Lifestyle and Longevity

Lifestyle and Longevity

Tom Taylor

Copyright © 2024 by Tom Taylor

All rights reserved. No part of this publication may be reproduced, distributed, or transmitted in any form or by any means, including photocopying, recording, or other electronic or mechanical methods, without the prior written permission of the copyright owner and the publisher, except in the case of brief quotations embodied in critical reviews and certain other noncommercial uses permitted by copyright law. For permission requests, write to the publisher, addressed "Attention: Permissions Coordinator," at the address below.

ARPress
45 Dan Road Suite 5
Canton MA 02021
Hotline: 1(888) 821-0229
Fax: 1(508) 545-7580

Ordering Information:
Quantity sales. Special discounts are available on quantity purchases by corporations, associations, and others. For details, contact the publisher at the address above.

Printed in the United States of America.

ISBN-13:   Paperback   979-8-89389-436-3
           eBook   979-8-89389-437-0

Library of Congress Control Number: 2024917386

I would like to dedicate the book to Joy

Contents

Chapter 1 : Introduction 1
Chapter 2 : Genetics 8
Chapter 3 : Epidemiology 10
Chapter 4 : Exercise and Longevity 13
Chapter 5 : Differences Between the Sexes 16
Chapter 6 : Diabetes 18
Chapter 7 : The Technological Revolution 24
Chapter 8 : The Impact of Television and
Social Media on Lifestyle 27
Chapter 9 : Alcohol. 28
Chapter 10 : Sources of Energy. 30
Chapter 11 : Obesity, the Major Killer 34
Chapter 12 : The Nature of Obesity 36
Chapter 13 : The Long-Term Hazards of Obesity. . . 39
Chapter 14 : The Psychology of the Obese State . . . 48
Chapter 15 : Nutritional Requirements. 53
Chapter 16 : Maintaining a Healthy Weight 55
Chapter 17 : Supermarkets: The Food We Buy 69
Chapter 18 : Dementia 72
Chapter 19 : Sleep 76
Chapter 20 : What to do in Retirement? 78
Chapter 21 : Drugs and Longevity 80

Chapter 22 : Deaths from Trauma 83
Chapter 23 : Suicide 85
Chapter 24 : The Unpredictable 87
Chapter 25 : Conclusions—The Bottom Line 90
Suggested Further Reading 94

CHAPTER 1
INTRODUCTION

I had a wonderful stress-free life up to the age of thirteen. My dad referred to me as the happiest guy alive. Then I awoke one morning to learn that Dad had a major heart attack and was in hospital, where he remained for six months, having a series of further heart attacks. He was somewhat overweight, having enjoyed my mother baking apple and custard pies. He also smoked, as did most of adult males in those days. He went home to die of a further heart attack when I was a student.

This experience changed my life and destroyed my sense of security. One thing it did for me was to make me study harder at school, as I'd decided that I wanted to study medicine. Many years later, I have spent my life performing surgery, doing research, and studying diet and obesity. I have performed over a thousand gastric bypasses for obesity and diabetes. We are still learning what the most important factors are in preventing heart disease, diabetes, vascular disease, and dementia, which are the major killers today and beginning to have such an impact as to start reducing longevity, despite evidence that exists for the potential of prolonging life much further.

Everyone is interested in longevity issues—it is life. Our major killers are all related to diet. "How can I influence my life expectancy, and at what price?" I am frequently asked. Statistically, there are numerous observations and scientific studies that point to factors that influence longevity. Many of them are real and actual; many are controversial. In Great Britain, for the first time in this century, life expectancy has fallen in both males and females. In contrast, there are more centenarians alive than ever before.

Between 1900 and 2000, life expectancy was extended from the mid-forties to the mid-seventies. This was the century when unprecedented, huge technological advances took place. For example, from most people using horse-drawn vehicles to now flying from New York to Australia in a day. For those living in Western countries, food became more available and plentiful, with around-the-year access to most foodstuffs becoming available. The first half of the century was punctuated by two world wars, each on a scale never previously encountered. These wars brought with them necessities leading to technical innovations that amounted to citizens ultimately having access to their own automobiles and international travel. Hard physical grafting became replaced by mechanical diggers, advanced agricultural implements, and motor-driven building tools, and with these the shift to a more sedentary lifestyle and types of employment.

The second half of the twentieth century brought about a revolution in medical care. In the early years, pneumonia and poliomyelitis were endemic, along with major outbreaks of infectious diseases like smallpox.

At the end of World War II there was only one breakthrough antibiotic—penicillin—no tissue transplantation, no open-heart surgery, no intensive care units, no chemotherapy, and no joint replacement. The medical innovations of this half century saved and prolonged the lives of millions, each of them adding huge costs to what is now the bottomless pit of present-day healthcare.

Probably the greatest innovation in healthcare in terms of saving lives was vaccination. Smallpox has been eliminated worldwide, deaths from polio no longer exist, and measles, rubella, and mumps have become rare diseases. There are, however, now new viral diseases that are highly lethal, such as HIV and Ebola. Influenza, though, to some extent protected against by vaccination, still presents a major threat to world health as a result of the mutations of the virus to new and more aggressive manifestations. We continually face the possibility of an outbreak of a new mutation of influenza that could kill millions. The outbreak of influenza at the end of the First World War affected one-third of the population of the world and killed more people than the war. The devastating mass fatalities of Covid-19 could not have been foreseen and there could be more fatalities from new viral diseases or mutations of existing viruses in the future. Covid destroyed the lives and lifestyles of millions from children to the elderly.

Not only have new vaccines had a huge effect, but other epidemiological studies have highlighted aspects of our lifestyles that have been shown to be a danger to health and longevity. The most notable of these was the discovery in the 1950s that smoking causes early death in millions as a result of lung cancer, vascular disease, heart disease, bronchitis, emphysema, and pneumonia. This discovery has led to social measures of public education, warning of the dangers, which has led to a massive reduction in smoking in society.

The major killer in the Western world remains cardiovascular disease, which includes coronary thrombosis, heart failure, and stroke. Open-heart surgery was developed in the late 1960s and early 70s, and its use has expanded exponentially. Hundreds of thousands of coronary bypass grafts have been performed with low morbidity and mortality and excellent long-term outcomes. Techniques of revascularizing the heart have now become minimally invasive, the arterial blockages being dilated and stented by passing instruments from a small incision in the groin or upper arm through the arterial system to the site of the disease. This is another area where public health studies on diet and smoking can make a huge impact from the point of view of disease prevention, and new drugs have had a major impact. More studies are required into strategies to promote the prevention of the disease. New advances in heart surgery, cancer treatments, and trauma surgery have been dependent upon the development of high-technology intensive care units with ventilators and active, aggressive supporting measures. These were developed in the early 1970s and have become progressively more advanced and sophisticated. Concurrently, chemotherapy for cancer has been developed and enhanced over the last fifty years, producing prolongation of life. Diseases such as breast cancer and other malignancies such as Hodgkin's disease and testicular cancer have been greatly impacted.

We have discovered that our major killing diseases are related to diet. It is now known that an appropriate diet can significantly contribute to the prevention and treatment of diseases, especially cancer, diabetes, cardiovascular disease, and dementia. Over the years, there has been much confusion in the advice and recommendations given in relation to diet. In the 1950s, animal fat was criticized and blamed as the major factor in contributing to our major killer, heart disease. It was later blamed for breast and colon cancer, as well as hypertension and stroke. Coffee consumption has been in and out of favor over recent decades for several disorders, including pancreatic cancer and heart disease. It is currently linked to prolonged longevity. Chocolate, also condemned in the past, has now been resurrected as a possible adjunct to avoiding heart disease. A recent study has shown that three bars of chocolate a month can reduce the chances and contribute to the management of heart failure. Research on more than half a million adults showed a 13% lower risk of heart failure in those eating chocolates compared with those who ate none.

Now the chief factors involved in the major killers—heart disease, stroke, hypertension, dementia, and obesity—are all related to the same dietary factors, and the major enemy is sugar. Over recent years there has been a marked increase in the deaths of young women in Western countries because they have adopted unhealthy lifestyles. They are succumbing largely to diseases hitherto more common in males. The countries where the most women aged between thirty and seventy years are dying of major diseases are the US (11.8%), the Netherlands (9.7%), Denmark (9.5%), and the United Kingdom (9%). This contrasts with Portugal, Italy, and Spain, where the incidence is less than 7%. Illnesses that cause the deaths of these younger ladies are diabetes, heart disease, cancer, and lung disease. Overall figures for Western men in this age range succumbing to these diseases is 13%. One factor is the increased amount of alcohol consumed by women, who now drink as much as men, and evidence shows that more men have stopped smoking than women. In contrast, deaths for Eastern women, where drinking and smoking are less common, is much lower at 5%.

Undoubtedly, women's recent lifestyle choices are the major contributors to the development of the above noncommunicable life threats. There is information available to us that can lead, in a relatively simple way, to avoiding, or at least deferring, the onset of today's killer diseases, and these are related to diet. In addition, there is a large amount of scientific evidence available that proves smoking is a major killer. Smoking tobacco is the worst thing you can do for your health.

Major factors in assessing the importance of various diets relate to the duration of studies and the reliability of the collected data. What did you eat yesterday? How many calories did you consume? How much did you drink? I have difficulty in remembering what I ate, how much, and how many calories were imbibed, and that is just in an extremely short term, let alone over many years. Many changes will obviously occur in most people's diets over the years of their life, and it is difficult to predict the timing and duration of exposure to the essential dietetic components. We can, however, look at environmental studies that identify some parts of the world where those residents, for all their lives and consequently eating the same diet, live for extraordinarily long periods of time. Numerous epidemiological studies have looked at the factors in locations where longevity appears to have been prolonged. Conversely, despite all of the many studies on diet and health problems associated with dietary indiscretion, weight gain, diabetes, heart disease, and stroke increased annually and are now causing, for the first time in over a century, a shortening of life expectancy.

We are, however, what we eat, and eating the correct diet in the long term can undoubtedly prolong longevity. The major question remains: what sort of diet should we eat, how much and how often, and what essential factors, such as exercise, go along with eating the right diet? We are also born with a predetermined set of genes from our parents, which are difficult, if not impossible, to change.

We have to form a long-term strategy. Life is not a hundredyard dash. It is a marathon, and preparation should be constructed over the decades in anticipation of the long term. It starts in early life, and "points" can be built up over successive decades. Type-II diabetes, totally related to dietary excess, is becoming prevalent in childhood, and suicide in early life is a growing problem.

Being healthy throughout life is important in staving off weight gain, joint problems, and conditions that are lifethreatening in later life. The healing diet should be a long-term, hopefully a lifelong policy, beginning at least in the twenties when junk food should be avoided and smoking strictly banned. Suicide is the leading cause of death in the twenties and thirties. In the thirties, weight gain tends to occur with decreasing exercise and slowing of the metabolism. Few Premier League footballers keep on playing for the top clubs after their early thirties. In the forties, the risk of serious health conditions, such as cancer and heart disease, start to increase. Women become subject to menopausal problems, and their bone health begins to be threatened. Problems beginning in the forties progress and further develop into the fifties, and cancer levels begin to rise. Heart attacks become the number-one cause of death among men aged over fifty. Screening programs for breast and colon cancers are very valuable. In the sixties, joint disease becomes prevalent and inhibits exercise and mobility. Blood pressure and cholesterol levels tend to climb, and the seventies herald a huge surge in dementia, which increases over subsequent years and is now possibly about to supersede vascular disease as the commonest cause of death.

There have been massive changes in lifestyle over the past century. Mankind has evolved over millions of years, but only in the last century has change developed at an unrelenting pace never before experienced. We have walked the roads to and from our destinations, day in, day out, for thousands of years. In the past few thousand years, the fastest mode of transport was the horse. In the past century, we have developed technologies enabling us to travel the world in a day, New York to Australia. We have also become dependent upon mechanization in every walk of life. Buses to school, cars to work, engines to dig and till the soil, to build roads, buildings, and manufactured goods. The effect of lying in front of a screen eating and drinking carbohydrate-laced foods created a new model of human. Our supermarket shelves are packed with cheap, mass-produced, good-tasting, readily available food that is packed with calories. These foods are constantly attractively displayed in the advertisements on the televisions to which the population has become glued.

Interestingly, people who migrate to the US from poor areas such as Latin America and Asia adopt these Western lifestyles and become obese. Improved nutrition has done much to enhance human performance, physical and possibly intellectual performance, but modern nutrition has also created syndrome X, which is killing thousands. Syndrome X is caused by the disturbance of body chemistry emanating from lack of exercise and the consumption of refined sugars. Think of a one-pound bag of refined sugar. Think of 150 bags in a pile. This is how much the average person eats per year. Cans of soda contain over two hundred calories per drink, all of which is sugar-refined carbohydrates. There is the equivalent of nine teaspoons of sugar in a can of Coke.

A recent study of nearly two million deaths has shown that longevity relates markedly to body mass index (BMI). A high body mass index relates to all major causes of death, as well as less common causes like kidney and liver failure and also suicide. The higher the BMI, the greater the impact on longevity. In addition, BMI levels below normal also reduce longevity, possibly as a result of poor nutrition. Maintaining a healthy weight is a lifelong delicate balance more easily achieved by some than others. Over thirty years, a daily excess intake of just seven calories over expenditure will produce a thirty-three-pound weight gain.

How can we improve the current public health situation? We are faced with the equivalent of mass extermination. Let's take a look at the evidence.

Chapter 2
Genetics

Genetics is the study of heredity and the variation of inherited characteristics. A gene is made of DNA, a complex double helix molecule that conveys basic genetic instructions. These instructions are used for making molecules and controlling chemical reactions. Genes are passed from parents to offspring, providing the basis of inheritance. Charles Darwin showed that individuals inherit a smooth blend of traits from their parents.

Genes undoubtedly have a major role to play in longevity. The evolutionary process has led to survival of the fittest, where genetic change has been largely responsible for the increase in longevity. Much of the thirty-year-plus extension of life expectancy achieved over the past century can be attributed to a number of non-genetic reasons. Genes, however, are responsible for a predetermined maximum range of survival. No man has ever lived for more than 115 years, and few reach their nineties. Centenarians are rare but exist more frequently in some communities than others; inherited factors are in part responsible for this. Alligators and some turtles can live for over two hundred years, and dogs live, on the whole, from ten to fifteen years due to genetic factors. If you feed or care for your dog however carefully, there is no way that it is going to live for more than twenty years, as this is a genetically programmed and determined parameter.

Throughout the evolutionary process, lifespan may slowly increase if there is a continuance in the production of healthy offspring. Diets can influence genetic stability and control, but probably by a very slow process. Conversely, sugar has been shown to increase aging in primitive organisms by activating the genes RAS and PKA.

By recently developed technology in genetic manipulation, simple organisms such as yeast can live up to five times longer, and certain crops can grow stronger and become more disease resistant. Despite our escalating knowledge of DNA and the potential to manipulate it, which now exists, so far we have been able to do nothing to influence longevity. However, genetic manipulation has recently been used to alter T-cells from the patient's own body, which are then reinjected and used to treat blood cancers. This is in its infancy and ultimately could be extended to the treatment of solid tumors, such as breast and lung cancer, and to potentially affect longevity. There is, therefore, a potential for gene manipulation to increase life expectancy.

Genes can play an important role in families that may have longer-living characteristics. Clearly, they are an overriding factor determining how long a species can expect to live. Chimpanzees have a sequence of DNA amounting to 95% of that in man, but they never live beyond the age of fifty. The behavior and control of genes that can influence longevity and disease requires more detailed study, and the technology is becoming available to achieve this. The challenges that face geneticists in resetting the genetically controlled timeclock are immense and currently in the remote future.

Chapter 3
Epidemiology

Epidemiology is the method used to find causes of health outcomes and diseases in populations. In epidemiology, the patient is the community, and individuals are viewed collectively. The definitive way of evaluating a medicine or method of treatment is by carrying out a randomized controlled clinical trial. This is virtually impossible in terms of assessing the roles of many factors, such as dietary differences, on longevity, as the periods of study would be too long to make a standard type of study feasible. However, accurate comparisons of long-and shorter-living communities can be made by looking at epidemiological studies. These can identify geographical areas where there are long-lived populations in stable communities and then look at the effect on their longevity if they move, long term, into a totally different environment.

When considering dietary differences, it is not only the content of the diet that is important but also the amount eaten. Mice and rats fed on low-calorie diets can live up to 40% longer. Longterm studies on monkeys have shown that those fed on a lowcalorie diet both live longer and are less prone to disease. Studies of long-living populations can be compared with other populations in the short term when dietary and other differences come to light and valuable data is accrued. Dietary factors, though fundamental, are not the only factors to be considered. There are people in Ecuador who are long-lived, probably as a result of genetic differences, and there are those in Mediterranean countries whose longevity depends upon diet. Indigenous genetic Italians living in areas in northern Italy live long lives, but Italians living in Chicago increase their incidence of Western diseases—diabetes, heart disease, stroke and obesity—when compared with the relatives who remain in Italy. They eat bacon, sausage, eggs, pasta, white bread, red meat, and cheese. Much of the food they eat is fried and taken with sugary drinks. Population studies show an association between longevity and a diet that is low in animal protein and rich in complex carbohydrates found in vegetables, olive oil, and legumes. Although excess sugar intake is the major cause of diabetes, high protein and saturated fat intake also predisposes to cancer and diabetes. A Mediterranean diet with high levels of olive oil and nuts is associated with reduced cardiovascular events and mortality. A previous boss of mine, Dr. Michael DeBakey, was very slim, ate little, and would frequently nibble nuts. He lived to the age of ninety-nine and worked right up to the end of his life.

When diets that reduce calorific intake by 20% or more are maintained in the long term, there is a risk of them affecting necessary metabolic processes, including wound healing, immune response, and cold temperature tolerance. Excess hair loss is an early sign of inadequate nutrition, so the maintenance of an adequate balanced diet needs to be kept throughout life.

Populations in Japan, Italy, California, and Ecuador, where there is a high prevalence of centenarians have undergone intense study. The Californian studies are particularly interesting, as there is a large racial mix, and people moving from other countries to California, such as second-generation Japanese, develop the disease pattern and comparative death rates as those of the indigenous Californian, which are different from those back in their own country. The difference in lifestyle can largely be attributed to dietary change. Those countries with long-lived populations share largely plant-based diets, which are relatively low in proteins, refined carbohydrates, and trans fats. They have a relatively low calorific intake, and obesity is virtually nonexistent.

In Okinawa, Japan, the long-lived population eats only onetenth of the amount of meat, eggs, and dairy products compared to the American diet, but they eat twice as many vegetables, three times as many grains, and ten times as much fish. This population also indulges in a lot of physical exercise. In long-lived Italian communities, evidence points to the eating of low-protein, highvegetable, and olive-oil-based diets, but there seems to be a beneficial effect from increasing protein intake in the advanced decades of life, as this preserves muscle power and mobility. Several areas in Italy exhibit marked longevity, and these all share a diet that is largely composed of lots of vegetables and wholemeal bread. Northern Italy has one of the highest proportions of centenarians worldwide. There is also an area in southern Italy that has one of the highest numbers of centenarians. Here they live on a low-protein, otherwise Mediterranean diet. In California, Adventists live an average of six to ten years longer than the average person and eat a diet that is rich in vegetables, legumes, and nuts.

The incidence of disease also varies widely in different parts of the world. In Okinawa, the incidence of breast cancer is onesixth, and prostate cancer one-seventh, that in the US. Native Greenlanders have lived traditionally on a diet that consists of meat and blubber from seals and whales. These mammals feed on fish whose flesh has a high concentration of omega-3 fatty acids. Heart disease is extremely rare in the classical indigenous Greenland natives. Several studies have shown that eating fish reduces death from heart disease.

Human size, strength, and mobility has continued to increase or improve year by year, as has, probably, intellectual ability. In 1954, Roger Bannister ran a mile in under four minutes, a barrier hitherto regarded as unachievable. Now, however, many middledistance runners consistently break the four-minute mile, and the record is down to three minutes and forty-three seconds. It is hard to know whether diet, training, genetics, or evolution is the major factor responsible for this.

Chapter 4
Exercise and Longevity

The importance of energy expenditure cannot be overstressed as a fundamental issue in contributing to good health throughout life. Physical inactivity is a major factor in contributing to the major killers. While increasing numbers, often many thousands in one center (as in London, New York, Houston), run marathons, far greater numbers refrain from indulging in any form of physical activity. Physical energy expenditure ranges from static functions, such as rapidly increasing and decreasing muscle tone, to voluntarily moving in athletic activity, as in running. The energy expenditure of minimal daily activity in a non-exercising person is about 50% greater than the basal metabolic rate, the latter being the amount of energy expenditure required to maintain the stability of an individual while totally resting, such as lying in bed all day. Moderately active individuals add approximately another 20% to this figure. Females tend to expend fewer calories by physical activity then do males. Obese individuals show a reduced variety of fine movements, such as moving around in the chair and gesticulating, than those of normal weight.

Day-to-day normal activities burn between 500 and 1,000 calories. Steady walking uses 300 calories per hour, cycling 400 calories, and running, rowing, and swimming 500 to 600 calories per hour. Continuous weightlifting, as in body pump, will expend up to 600 calories per hour and raises the body's energy expenditure over the next six to eight hours, up to an excess of a further 600 calories above the basal level.

The effects of physical exercise in relation to total energy turnover each day are relatively small. It is unlikely that many will exercise for more than one hour per day, therefore increasing their resting energy of two thousand calories by more than an additional six hundred calories. Exercise is excellent for health and as part of a diet treatment regime, but it doesn't contribute as much as reduced food intake to weight loss. It should be part of the dietary regime, and as such is a useful aid to weight reduction in maintaining a healthy body weight.

Most studies that place emphasis on exercise experience a high attrition rate, even when the program lasts for only a few weeks or months. The harder the exercise program, the greater is the rate of attrition. Gymnasiums tend to take more money from members who don't attend rather than those who use them regularly.

It is possible that the decrease in activity that occurs with aging may form the basis for the decline in muscle mass and lean body mass as people grow older. Replacement of lean tissue by fat associated with aging worsens the problem of energy imbalance, since the basal need for energy falls with the total reduction of metabolically active lean tissue. This will lead to a further drop in basal metabolic rate and a tendency to gain inert body fat.

Exercise is good for the cardiovascular system, particularly that which increases the heart rate. Regular exercise is important in old age and tends to improve a person's psychology and sense of well-being, probably by the production of endorphins. Energy expenditure does not in itself increase muscle mass, though weightlifting, along with protein intake, will do this. Exercise helps to maintain lean body mass. Not only are the effects of aerobic exercise positive, but working with weights increases the ratio of body protein to body fat, which is beneficial, and this also stimulates metabolic activity. Exercise is also good for the brain. In addition, exercise tends to improve the immune system, which otherwise weakens with age.

It is important to exercise throughout life, particularly with advancing age. It helps with weight reduction but is not as major a factor as dietary restraint. However massively exhausting running a marathon is, it burns about three thousand calories, less than what is eaten in a large Thanksgiving dinner.

Lack of exercise is an important factor in the obesity equation. The less walking a person does in his day-to-day activities, the more likely he is to be overweight. Exercise increases academic performance, assertiveness, confidence, emotional stability, independence, memory, mood, sexual satisfaction, and well-being. In addition, exercise programs decrease anger, anxiety, depression, and even alcohol abuse. Exercise programs are selected by those who are relatively fit. Obese people, for example, are often opposed to exercise programs. They are self-conscious, lacking in self-esteem, and frequently have difficulty performing the requisite exercises because they are carrying so much extra fat that they may be restricted by breathlessness, joint pains, and just difficulty in dealing with the excess weight. Many morbidly obese patients are too disabled to exercise or even climb a flight of stairs. Those who join exercise programs are frequently soon disillusioned by the slow results achieved and the fact that a can of Coca-Cola contains more calories than those expended in a thirty-minute exercise schedule.

The importance of exercise cannot be over emphasized. It is important in preventing heart attacks, strokes, and the development of diabetes. Exercise does not necessarily increase hunger. In fact, a thirty to forty-minute walk, by virtue of giving an endorphin drive, can lead to a suppression of appetite. Also, the results of participating in an exercise program are a disincentive for the subject to then go home and eat excessive amounts of food.

Finally, exercise not only burns calories but tends to increase basal metabolic rate, giving rise to a further erosion of the calorie load taken in. Another useful manifestation of exercise is that it stimulates muscle production and converts fat into muscle. Additionally, the endorphin drive produced by exercise results in a feeling of well-being that enables people to adopt a more positive attitude to life and its problems.

Chapter 5
Differences Between the Sexes

All studies have shown that females tend to live longer than males. The disease distribution, though not their prevalence, are the same. One in eight women will develop breast cancer, and a large proportion of elderly males will suffer from prostate cancer, though the mortality from this is less than that from breast cancer in females. There are identifiable differences between the sexes, but the major killers tend to be consistent throughout the male and the female populations.

Living to the ripe old age of ninety depends upon body size, height, and weight, as well as the level of physical activity, which seems to influence a woman's lifestyle more than it does that in a man. A recent study showed that women who live to ninety were, on average, taller and had put on less weight from the age of twenty as compared to women who were shorter and heavier. No such association was seen for men. However, men saw more benefit from physical activity than women.

In 1986, researchers asked over seven thousand Norwegian men and women between the ages of fifty-five and sixty-nine about their height, current weight, and their weight at the age of twenty. Both genders also told researchers about their current physical activity levels, which included walking, gardening, home improvement, biking, and sports. The men and women were then sorted into daily activity quotas: less than thirty minutes, thirty to sixty minutes, and ninety minutes or more. The groups were monitored until they died or reached the age of ninety. Of the 7,807 participants, 433 men and 994 women lived to that age. Issues that could affect longevity, such as current or past smoking and the level of alcohol use, were also taken into consideration.

Men and women in the study fared very differently when it came to the impact of body size and exercise. Women who weighed less at the age of twenty and put on less weight as they aged were more likely to live longer than heavier women. Height was a major factor; the study found women who were taller than five feet nine were 31% more likely to live into their nineties than women who were less than five feet three. Neither height nor weight seemed to factor into whether the men reach their nineties, but activity level did.

Men who spent ninety minutes or more being active were 39% more likely to live to ninety than men who were physically active for less than thirty minutes per day. In addition, for each thirty minutes a day the men were active, they were 5% more likely to reach that age.

In contrast, women who were physically active for more than sixty minutes a day were only 21% more likely to live to ninety than those who did thirty minutes or less, and beyond the former there was no bonus for increasing activity. The study found that the optimal exercise or activity level for females was sixty minutes per day.

CHAPTER 6
DIABETES

Diabetes is a chronic metabolic disorder that leads to abnormally high concentrations of blood sugar. It is caused by the inadequate production of insulin by the pancreas. There are two main types of diabetes: type 1 and type 2. In type 1, the immune system destroys the cells of the pancreas, which makes insulin. Type 2 diabetes is most frequently associated with obesity, and over time insulin resistance develops.

In 2015, 30.3 million people in the United States, or 9.4% of the population, had diabetes, and the disease affects one in four people over the age of sixty-five. Risk factors for the development of type 2 diabetes, which applies to over 90% of sufferers of obesity, are physical inactivity, genetic factors, race, and high blood pressure. Diabetes is a bad disease to have and can lead to such problems as heart disease, stroke, kidney failure, eye problems leading to blindness, dental disease, nerve damage producing loss of sensation and difficulty walking, and vascular problems such as gangrene.

We are experiencing an epidemic of diabetes, which is triggering over one million cases of heart disease annually. This is producing heart failure, heart attacks, angina, and strokes, which are linked to unhealthy lifestyles. About half of the strokes are fatal, and one-third of the patients with heart failure will die within a year. Children as young as nine are now suffering from diabetes. It is now considered to be the fastest growing health crisis of its time. The overall cost of treatment is about $50 billion per year. About one-third of cases of heart disease and one-fifth of all strokes are linked to diabetes. Type 2 diabetes is largely preventable through diet and exercise. Those with diabetes are about four times more likely to have a heart attack or stroke. Men and women aged between thirty-five and sixty-four with type 2 diabetes are much more likely to die prematurely compared with those without this condition. Those with type 1 diabetes, which is not linked to diet or obesity, are three to four times as likely to die prematurely. Patients with type 2 diabetes have a 30% higher chance of being diagnosed with cancer, and they have a far worse survival rate. Women have a 31% higher risk; for men, the increased risk is 22%.

Thirteen types of cancer in diabetics are increased compared with the normal population, including breast, bowel, and liver; these are associated with obesity. The incidence of lung and skin cancer, which are unrelated to obesity, are also increased in diabetics. The findings suggest that diabetes itself is directly related to cancer risk, which scientists believe could be because high blood sugar levels cause DNA damage that predisposes to malignancies. Obesity-related cancers are at their highest risk with diabetic men. They have an 84% increased risk of dying from these cancers; in women, the increase is 48%. For cancers unrelated to obesity, cancer deaths are increased in diabetics by 18% for women, 5% for men. A study on half a million diabetics showed a 231% increased risk of liver cancer, 119% pancreatic, 30% lung, and 20% bladder cancer. These findings underscore the importance of more active prevention and treatment of diabetes. Research has shown that fasting can reduce the risk of cancer by cutting weight and insulin levels. Intermittent fasting causes the body to switch energy sources from glucose to fat cells, which can stimulate activity in the brain. The food industry has not acted by the reformulation of fast-food products. The introduction of firm regulation to cut the sugar and fat content of food and the reduction in advertising fast junk food is urgently required.

Ancient man, for many thousands of years, ate unrefined carbohydrates as part of the hunter-gatherer type of diet. With these diets, the pancreas was stimulated to a much lesser extent than with present-day diets. Until two hundred years ago, humans ate less than one pound of refined sugars per year. Now, as stated, 150 pounds are eaten per year.

Sugar manufacturers, cola producers, and the packaged food industry have paved the way to the current situation. It might be said that sugar manufacturers have contributed to more deaths than all wars combined. We now eat increased amounts of carbohydrates in the form of simple sugars. All carbohydrates are broken down to simple sugars, mainly glucose. Glucose maintains the blood sugar at a steady level in the nondiabetic. Only the small amount of six hundred grams of carbohydrates are stored in the liver, and a little is stored in muscle. Any remaining glucose is converted to and stored as fat.

Complex starches found in vegetables are absorbed less rapidly and are slowly broken down to glucose, which protects the blood level of glucose from rising rapidly. It is the rapid absorption of ingested refined carbohydrates that increases the blood sugar concentration and stimulates insulin secretion. Healthy people secrete about twenty-five to thirty units of insulin per day from the pancreas. Insulin sweeps glucose into cells, where it is stored. Insulin prevents the level of glucose in the blood from rising. Too much insulin can produce dangerously low levels of blood sugar, leading to loss of consciousness and possibly death.

Production and utilization of insulin is the key to diabetes, as it allows sugars to enter the cells and provide energy. When the lock is faulty, sugars cannot enter the cells. They build up in the bloodstream, causing damage. Carrying excess fat in the body adds to the difficulty that insulin has in doing its job. If circulating sugar cannot enter the cells, the pancreas goes on pumping out more and more insulin. Ultimately, the excess insulin production may overshoot the mark and produce a marked fall in blood sugar concentration, which causes powerful appetite stimulation and weight gain.

Diabetics whose blood sugar is poorly controlled are continuously pouring out insulin, to which they become increasingly resistant. The high levels of blood sugar damages other organs, in particular the eye and the kidney, leading to blindness and renal failure. Extremes of blood sugar concentration, both low and high, can lead to coma, which is life-threatening. Diabetics also have a marked tendency to develop accelerated arteriosclerosis.

Excessive glucose intake over time produces insulin resistance. There is then a decrease in responsiveness, wherein fat cells, liver cells, and muscle cells become insensitive to insulin and blood glucose concentrations rise. Insulin resistance is a major factor in the development of obesity. The high levels of circulating insulin cause the body to store as much fat as possible, and resistance also leads to high blood pressure, heart disease, and stroke. A significant reduction of sugar intake will lower peak insulin levels and ultimately reduce insulin resistance.

The precise reasons why insulin resistance occurs are not fully known. Insulin resistance can run in families and is exacerbated by poor diet and unhealthy lifestyles, particularly smoking and drinking. Type 2 diabetes responds well to lifestyle changes, and in most cases will respond to dietary change, increased exercise, and weight loss. It is almost entirely preventable, but nonetheless the incidence has doubled in twenty years and is predicted continually to rise in the foreseeable future.

In the bloodstream, insulin converts sugars into minute fat particles called triglycerides. This causes fat storage, arteriosclerosis, coronary artery disease, peripheral vascular disease, and stroke. Triglycerides and cholesterol in high concentrations in the bloodstream are the main predictive factors for arteriosclerosis. There are two types of cholesterol: high density and low-density lipoprotein cholesterol, referred to as HDL and LDL.

High density lipoprotein cholesterol is good cholesterol, being protective, and low-density lipoprotein cholesterol is bad cholesterol and is the major factor in causing damage to the vascular system. The process of arteriosclerosis, or hardening of the arteries, still the major killer, begins with the deposition of streaks or plaques of yellowish-gray cholesterol on the lining of blood vessels. Over time, these plaques become raised and hard, narrowing crucial blood vessels and leading to thrombosis or complete blockage of the blood vessels. When this process occurs in the coronary arteries, it leads to angina and severe pain in the central chest, which sometimes radiates to the neck and arm. The pain results from the lack of blood supply to the muscle of the heart and the death of this essential muscle. Ultimately, the coronary arteries may become completely occluded. This is a condition known as coronary thrombosis, which cuts off the blood supply to the heart muscle. This condition, also referred to as myocardial infarction, remains the largest killer in Western civilization today. The strongest predictive factor for arteriosclerosis is hyperinsulinism.

Another problem associated with hyperinsulinism and high blood glucose levels is hypertension, or high blood pressure. Most cases of hypertension are attributed to hyperinsulinism, and this usually precedes the overtly diabetic state, sometimes referred to as prediabetes. Hypertension, in itself, predisposes to coronary artery disease, stroke, and kidney failure.

For many years, the philosophy about the ill effects of ingested fat prevailed. Fifty years ago, the main villain in producing the rapidly increasing wave of heart attacks and strokes was thought to be animal fat. Prior to 1900, coronary thrombosis was rare. There is now, however, an increasing amount of evidence that unsaturated nontrans fats are good for us. These are not necessarily the fats in margarine; they are fats like olive oil and those in avocados.

As mentioned in Chapter 3, it has long been known that Mediterranean races have a much lower incidence of coronary artery disease and stroke than in northern Europeans. This may be related to a diet rich in unsaturated fats that contain omega-3 fatty acids. A commonly referenced study, the Lyons heart study, looked at the influence of a butter substitute, canola oil, which is a monosaturated fat with omega-3 fatty acids. In a series of patients, all of whom had previously had a heart attack, there was a 70% decrease in subsequent heart attacks in those who received the good fats. Another study, the Gissi prevention trial, showed that fish oil capsules containing omega-3 fatty acids decreased sudden deaths from heart attacks and strokes. Omega-3 fatty acids, therefore, plentiful in fish, seemed to confer some protection against the development of heart attacks and strokes.

Omega-3 fatty acids in large doses are also effective in treating depression. Additionally, a number of studies have shown that nuts, which contain a lot of unsaturated fats, are protective against heart attacks and strokes.

Good fats are essential fatty acids that fall into two main categories: omega-3 and the omega-6 groups. Omega-3 fatty acids are found in leaves and plant seeds, egg yolks, and in salmon, herring, cod, tuna, and mackerel. Omega-6 fatty acids are found in plant seeds, especially black currents. In addition, there are omega-9 fatty acids, the most plentiful of which, oleic acid, is found in olive oil, some nuts, and avocados.

The American Heart Association has for many years stated that eating saturated fats such as butter and lard will accelerate the process of arteriosclerosis and lead to clogging of the arteries and thrombosis. Conversely, eating foods high in polyunsaturated fats was thought to keep the arteries clear. Robert Atkins, well known for the Atkins diet, came out in strong defiance of the above dictum, advocating eating a diet high in fat and protein. Perhaps ironically, Atkins died of a heart attack while jogging. Even the famous long-standing and most-often quoted study, the Framingham study, realized that there was uncertainty surrounding the above recommendations. Supporting Atkins position, Cestelli has stated, "We found that the people who ate the most cholesterol, or the most saturated fat, or even the most calories from fat, weighed the least and were physically the most active."

In marked contrast, there is much evidence that the widely used cholesterol lowering drugs, the statins, can radically reduce deaths from coronary artery disease, and huge numbers of the population take these prophylactically. The modern American diet produces a serious imbalance in the ratio of omega-3 to omega-6 fatty acids. This is a result of consuming a lot of refined corn, soy, sunflower, and canola oils, which contain large amounts of omega6 fatty acids and relatively small amounts of omega-3 fatty acids. In contrast, for centuries, the source of essential fatty acids was omega-3 rich whole grains, nuts, vegetables, and egg yolks.

The combined evidence to date raises serious questions about the role of dietary saturated fats in causing heart disease and the supposed role of polyunsaturated fats in preventing it. It is argued that all people over the age of sixty-five would benefit from a reduction in cholesterol produced by statins, even if they have a normal cholesterol concentration in their blood. This would result in a reduction of fatal heart attacks and strokes, and the cost of the statin drugs is now very low.

Chapter 7
The Technological Revolution

Modern humans developed between 100,000 and 150,000 years ago, coincidental with the development of controlled agriculture. A steady and predictable source of food, which could be replenished through the seasons, led to the development of large population centers. The shift of wild animal meat and vegetation to cultivated grains deprived humans of many of the essential amino acids, vitamins, and minerals, which they had continued to thrive on for over three million years. Although the lifespan increased at this time, average height diminished.

Nutritional deficiencies started to manifest themselves in skeletal remains, dental cavities developed, and bacterial infections increased, many of them life-threatening. Obesity, however, was not a problem. This remained the situation until approximately a hundred years ago when the technological revolution led to a reduced need for hard physical labor. Mechanization replaced digging by hand; all the early canals were dug out by labor, using shovels. Improved technology has made crops of grain and dairy products cheaper to produce and more plentiful. Along with these changes has come the bubble of obesity, produced by sugars, fast food, and lack of exercise, which is now leading to a reduction in life expectancy for the first time in thousands of years. This change in lifestyle has brought about and coincided with marked socioeconomic changes.

In the United States, high-income people tend to be thinner than those of lower socioeconomic status. One in three adults living below the poverty line is obese, compared with one in six in households with an income in excess of $70,000 per year. In addition, over one in three African Americans is obese, and obesity markedly reduces their life expectancy as, with reduced income, they are eating the wrong foods.

The reasons underlying the above are not altogether clear. It does not appear entirely to be a simple question of eating fast food instead of a healthier diet. Processed foods are not just cheap; they are tasty, attractive, and filling. People preferred burgers over healthy eating. A significant problem is that, calorically, the best value for money is food high in refined carbohydrate content, and people eating it are not aware of the significant effect it can have on their longevity. Education is important, but the other important factor is that lean fish and steak is much more expensive than McDonald's hamburgers.

The tasty attraction of the wrong foods is particularly prevalent in children. Children, particularly, are prone to eat the wrong foods. They have little money and their parents may be out at work. Consequently, they go to the corner store and buy junk foods, which they eat in front of the televisions on which these colorful and tasty products have been attractively advertised.

Advertising has an influence on life expectancy. The power of advertising cannot be underestimated. We are all vulnerable to the effects produced by the advertising world. Otherwise, companies would not spend such huge amounts on it. Look at the cost of advertisements shown during the Super Bowl, the program with the highest audience volume on television. One of the implications of this has been the provision of larger portions of food in restaurants. More people are using restaurants all the time. Only about 20% of the retail price in a restaurant relates to food. Therefore, it is not expensive to increase the amount of food given to the consumer. Most of the costs go to paying staff and rent. Advertising supersized meals at a bargain price is a major factor in successful marketing. Unfortunately, this results in overeating, a stretching of the stomach, and subsequently the desire to eat more with each meal. A vicious cycle develops so that, ultimately, the consumer, whether in a restaurant or at home, becomes used to eating much larger meals.

Portion size is important. An increase can result in a rise in intake of up to five hundred calories with each meal. Along with the bargain binge of fast food is a marked increased tendency to eat in restaurants. Approximately 50% of food budgets are now spent in restaurants. Wherein, in order to make the supersized meals tastier and more attractive, additional fats and carbohydrates are added. Unfortunately, the kind of fat that is used here has a high trans fatty acid concentration, and the carbohydrate glucose is hugely present. French fries, bread, pastry, and mayonnaise are among the items high in bad trans fatty acids.

An important factor that led to the huge growth in restaurants and the consumption of more fast foods by children has been the increasing tendency for both parents to be engaged in full-time employment. Under such circumstances, incomes are higher, women earn more, and there is no need to come home to cook after a full day's work. The result, therefore, has been to consume more fast food, as illustrated by the massive growth in the number of restaurants like McDonald's.

CHAPTER 8
THE IMPACT OF TELEVISION AND SOCIAL MEDIA ON LIFESTYLE

Prior to 1900, most houses were lit by candles or small oil lights. The development of electricity affected everyone's lifestyle. Electric lights extended the day by several hours; northern latitudes had hitherto experienced few hours of daylight in midwinter. Methods of heating were poor, restricted to coal and wood fires, which frequently needed refilling or stoking, and they went out at night. Electric lighting and electric power for heating and locomotion radically changed things and provided the more definitive changes of radio and television.

After World War II, the biggest change in Western life was due to the development of television. This was followed by the latest innovation, social media, with telephones and the Internet. Sitting in front of television sets in centrally heated apartments changed eating habits radically, but not for the better. The TV dinner has become predominant on the menu as more now gather around this, the center of the home. Television advertising has been exploited by the food industry, encouraging children to eat more sugared cereals and sweets, and tempting adults to indulge in double cheeseburgers, chips, multiple snacks, and alcohol. Advertising has changed American's lives, showing a new face, big, affluent and carefree, untouched by war or want.

After the war, cars became oversize, sporting big fins and capacious seats. In the new and rapidly expanding supermarket, colorful food packages promised more for your money. Restaurants served big steaks on bigger plates. With the addition of huge salads, this led to Americans learning to overeat long before the crisis of today.

Chapter 9
Alcohol

According to the US National Survey on Drug Use and Health, 86.4% of people aged eighteen or older reported drinking some alcohol—70.1% in the last year and 56% in the last month. Some, 28.9%, reported that they indulged in binge drinking in the last month. Approximately 88,000 deaths occur in each year in the United States due to alcohol. Those who died directly from an alcohol-related cause shortened their life expectancy by an average of thirty years. During the eighteen years of the Brezhnev regime in the USSR, life expectancy in males fell by ten years, the major cause being alcohol related. More than 7% of the American population over eighteen years of age has a drink problem. This is nearly 13.8 million Americans, and 8.1 million of them are alcoholics.

In the UK, the number of deaths linked to drinking rose by 6% in 2017, with 5,800 deaths in that year alone. This comes despite recent trends showing the nation turning its back on heavy drinking. Between 2011 and 2017, the number of people drinking more than fourteen units per week fell from 34% to 28% with men and from 18% to 14% with women.

Interestingly, drinking overall has significantly fallen among younger people, but binge drinking has increased, more in girls than boys. In total, 11% of girls aged 11 to 15 had been drunk in the last four weeks, compared with 7% for boys, statistics from 2016 show.

The statistics from the NHS in Great Britain shows that in 2017 to 2018, 338,000 people were admitted to hospital where the main cause was alcohol related, an increase from 293,000 in the years 2007 to 2008. In total 70% of admissions involved people over the age of forty-five. A total of 1.17 million hospital admissions in the NHS involved an alcohol-related condition that was either the main reason for admission or a secondary diagnosis.

Concern over these figures is being expressed by politicians who have suggested increasing the price and limiting the availability of alcohol and its advertising. More alcohol is now consumed in the home rather than in public houses because of the increased prices and the drinking-and-driving laws. Alcohol that is comprehensively displayed in all supermarkets is much less expensive than in public houses. One can counter these arguments by saying that the majority of people in England are drinking at, or within, very low risk levels.

Alcohol-related hospital admissions have risen by 15% in the past decade, amid warnings that drinking by baby boomers is taking its toll. The official statistics show that those aged 55 to 64 are now most likely to be admitted to hospital because of alcohol related diseases and injuries, followed by those aged 45 to 54 and those aged 65 to 74.

Alcohol-impaired driving fatalities accounted for 29% of total vehicle traffic fatalities in 2017. Between 1991 and 2017, the rate of drunk driving fatalities per hundred thousand population has decreased by 46% in the US and 68% among those are under twenty-one. The total fatalities from motor vehicle accidents has declined by only 16%. Among persons under twenty-one, drunk driving fatalities have decreased by 8%. According to the National Highway Traffic Safety Administration, 37,133 people died in traffic crashes in 2017 in the US. This included an estimated 10,874 people who were killed in drunk driving crashes involving a driver with an illegal blood alcohol concentration. Of these drivers, 68% were over twice the legal limit. In 2017, the drunk driving fatality rate was 3.4 per hundred thousand population nationally. In twenty-six states, the drunk driving fatality rate was at or below the national level. This reduction is possibly because of better education and increased law enforcement in relation to drinking and driving.

Chapter 10
Sources of Energy

The father of modern physics, Sir Isaac Newton, stated that energy cannot be created or destroyed but only converted from one form to another. Energy exists in many different forms, oil, coal, wind, the sun, and food. Burning the energy provided by food is essential for life. It permits us to run, walk, talk, and carry out our many lifetime activities.

Man derives his energy from three sources: proteins, carbohydrates, and fat. The body is an extremely efficient machine in the collection, storage, and utilization of energy, much more so than planes or cars. The energy taken in food is either used or stored. In the process of staying alive, maintaining our body structure and temperature, we utilize energy in the range of 1,500 to 2,000 calories per day. Overall, we utilize about 2,000 calories per day for women and 3,000 for men. Any energy that your body does not burn, it stores. Protein and carbohydrates provide four calories per gram; fat, nine calories per gram. Excess calorific intake is stored as fat.

In carbohydrate metabolism, the gut rapidly breaks down complex sugars into simple ones, predominantly glucose, fructose, and galactose. Sugars are absorbed through the small intestine and transported to the liver. Some of the glucose remains in the circulation to maintain the blood sugar at a constant level. It is transported into cells to provide energy. Glucose is broken down inside the cells by a process of glycolysis.

About 40% of calories in the average Western diet are derived from fat. Fats and oils are tri-esters of glycerol and various fatty acids. The ability of lipids to be stored in the body as fat provides a source for continuous energy production. Fats are used once carbohydrate stores have been depleted, which is normally after a period of about twelve hours of starvation. Absorption of lipids depends upon their being mixed with bile, and then they can be absorbed in the small intestine and converted to triglycerides, which are transported via the lymphatic system or directly into the bloodstream. Fat is used to form an essential component of cell membranes. A reduction in carbohydrate intake causes an increase in the breakdown of triglycerides and free fatty acids. Virtually all tissues, except the brain, require lipids as an energy source. When excessive amounts of lipids are metabolized and used for energy, breakdown products such as acetic acid give rise to a debilitating condition known as ketosis.

The main function of protein is to provide the building blocks for cells. Proteins can be utilized as a final source of energy in times of stress. Protein molecules taken in the diet are broken down by digestive enzymes into peptides and amino acids. These are the basic constituents of all larger protein molecules. There is a high turnover of body protein, and many grams of protein are carried through the body per hour. Amino acids are linked to cellular proteins and stored. Once the cell is replete, unused excess amino acids are converted into keto acids. A breakdown product of amino acids is ammonia, which in large amounts is toxic and depresses brain function. Protein is essential for production of the nucleic acids, DNA and RNA. These are the key to the fundamental genetic structure of man.

The body does not act as a storage organ for protein. Weightlifters store some energy in their increased muscle mass, but not a lot. Likewise, the body stores little carbohydrate, only about six hundred calories in the liver, the equivalent of two hours of exercise. Remaining calories are stored as fat. The fat stores are extremely efficient, and they have the potential to be huge, never being replete.

The morbidly obese person does not have a frame size much different than that of a skinny person. They have the same amount of bone, a little more muscle, the same size brain, lungs, guts, and heart. If the basic frame of a man who weighs 600 pounds is 150 pounds, he is carrying 450 pounds of fat and carrying it 24 hours a day—every time he moves, every time he walks, every time he climbs stairs. That is the equivalent of carrying about four large sacks of grain on his back. These "sacks of grain" strain the heart, the lungs, the muscles, and the joints.

Excess calories are rapidly converted into fat, because they cannot be lost if they are not burned, as fat contains nine calories per gram. An excess calorie intake over needs of a thousand calories per day, will lead to a weight gain of approximately a hundred grams per day, or two pounds per week. Not much? Well, two pounds per week is a hundred pounds per year. An excess of a thousand calories per day amounts to four cans of soda or four relatively small chocolate bars. And remember, it takes over two hours of cycling to burn it off. Consequently, just a little in excess of one's needs can have serious consequences leading to disease and early death.

Eating our way through mountains of sugar is the primary cause of heart attacks, vascular disease, strokes, and diabetes. Other related health problems that ensue are: breast and colon cancer, liver damage, increased tendency to thrombosis, and depression of the immune system. These disorders are those of the twentieth century, those of modern living. Coronary artery disease, stroke, and diabetes were all rare in the nineteenth century. Admittedly, many people died at a younger age, often of infectious diseases that today respond to antibiotics or may have been eradicated by vaccination.

Historically, much lip service was paid to the low-fat diet; the philosophy was one of avoiding fat and giving carte blanche to the increasing ingestion of carbohydrates. This has now been turned around by diets such as the low-or-no-carbohydrate Atkins diet. Sugar is the enemy, and sugar is toxic.

Sugar is an easily absorbed, pleasant to eat, and an inexpensive source of energy. Its bad effects are due to excessive stimulation of insulin, which causes excess fat storage and inhibits breakdown of previously stored fat. In addition, insulin signals our livers to make cholesterol and causes fatty infiltration of the liver. Diabetics have significantly higher total cholesterol and triglycerides in the blood than is normal.

Counting carbs has become a powerful fixture in the economy, as it has in society. Thousands of new low-carbohydrate foods and beverages hit the grocery shelves every year. All foods are now labeled with their energy content, which is useful. This has had a major effect on the food giants, as carb watching is here for the long term and is being legally enforced. It is possible that the effects of carb counting are beginning to become established as the population is repeatedly informed of the dangers of too much sugar.

After many consecutive years of weight gain, the American public has, in the last three or four years, shown a reduction in overweight adults by about 2%. In parallel, the number of orders in fast-food restaurants has risen by 12%, while in them consumption of French fries has fallen by 10%, and the national potato production has fallen by 5%.

Chapter 11
Obesity, the Major Killer

Obesity is the huge problem that underlies the major killers, heart disease, stroke, hypertension, and cancer. The word obesity refers to an excess of body fat. This is defined scientifically as a BMI of 30 kg/m² or in excess of 25% of the ideal body weight. Some forty million adults in the United States are obese by this definition. Of these, 7.5 million have a BMI of over 40 kg/m²; these suffer from severe or morbid obesity, the risks of which are life-threatening. This number has doubled in the last ten years and continues to increase rapidly. This is the major threat to longevity today.

Rates of obesity are increasing among Americans of all ages, ethnicities, and socioeconomic groups, including children. Presently, these rates are highest among African Americans, Hispanics, and lower socioeconomic groups. One of the most alarming statistics is that one in six American children between the ages of 6 and 19 are now obese. Prior to the millennials, during the last decade of the twentieth century, two million teenagers and young adults joined the ranks of the clinically obese. The vast majority of these have stayed there over the next two decades. Americans spend $40 billion per year on diets and weight-reducing methods. The annual medical costs related to obesity are over $75 billion. The cost of time lost from work as a direct result of obesity amounts to an additional $50 billion per year. The publicity surrounding this has had very little impact on the underlying problem.

The United States is a very body-conscious country whose public face, as depicted on magazine covers, in movies, and on television, is of youth, vitality, and sexual attractiveness. In reality, however, fewer and fewer Americans resemble this hallmark. Obesity will overtake smoking as the leading preventable cause of cancer in women in the next twenty years. Rising obesity levels, combined with falling smoking rates, will see these two causes switch places by 2040. Women are prone to more obesity-related cancers than men, including breast and womb cancer. Decades of effort into educating the public of the health risks of smoking, along with strong political action, including increasing taxation on tobacco and restriction of its use indoors, has paid off. Just as there is still increasing inducement for people to quit smoking, we need to act vigorously to halt the tide of obesity and with it weight-related cancers.

Currently, smoking causes about 12% of cancer cases in women, while excess weight is blamed for about 10%. While overall more males are overweight than females, more women are morbidly obese, and women are at risk because of its links to some particular cancers. Being overweight increases the risk of thirteen types of cancer, including bowel, liver, and kidney. One in ten breast cancer cases and one in three cancers of the womb are now linked to obesity.

In the industrial era, hard physical labor and periodic economic privation discouraged weight gain. Only the privileged leisure class had the opportunity to grow fat. Protective genetic traits that once defended the hearty from starvation now make those same persons susceptible to becoming overweight. At the same time, many people remain immersed in the socioeconomic issues of their families of origin. Where unlimited access to food and plumpness were once commonly associated with success and prosperity, now the reverse is true. Today, the car and the computer rule our lives, thrusting the majority to a leisure class that lacks physical activity and has a relatively unlimited access to food.

Chapter 12
The Nature of Obesity

Measuring the exact amount of fat in the body is difficult and can be inaccurate. X-ray and electrical methods are complex and unreliable. The most commonly used measure of obesity, the body mass index, is the weight in kilograms divided by the square of the height in meters.

Obesity is more than a cosmetic problem; it is the direct cause of a host of medical problems that are the biggest killers in Western society today. The triad of high blood pressure, high blood cholesterol, and diabetes is largely due to obesity. This trio is often referred to as syndrome X. Seventeen million Americans suffer from syndrome X, components of which are related and directly linked to excess sugar intake and insulin resistance. This collection of problems, rather than any single entity, now represents the number-one public health initiative facing Western society. This disorder is much more common than cancer and AIDS. It is the reason why we have created a new constellation of killer diseases from which everyone suffers to a variable degree.

It is our current lifestyle and behavior that is largely responsible for this problem. Today's lifestyle is sedentary, watching television, sitting in front of computers, and driving everywhere. The syndrome now affects not only the elderly or the middle-aged; it is having a major effect on children and teenagers.

People who migrate to the United States from poor areas such as Latin America and parts of Asia adopt Western lifestyles and become obese. Improved nutrition has done much to enhance human physical and intellectual performance, but modern nutrition has also created syndrome X, killing millions. Syndrome X is caused by a disturbance of body chemistry emanating from a lack of exercise and the consumption of refined carbohydrates.

The common gastrointestinal conditions that surgeons treat today are all self-induced by high sugar and low fiber diets. Gallstones, pancreatitis, diverticular disease, appendicitis, colon cancer, and hemorrhoids are all extremely rare in central Africa where a diet high in fiber and refined carbohydrates is prevalent. Take the central African out of his own environment and put him into the United States, however, and he will soon develop the same disorders as those of the indigenous Americans.

Our earliest ancestors probably ate foods that were similar to those eaten by apes and monkeys. These were fruits, shoots, nuts, tubers, and other vegetation found in the forests of Africa. Most of these plants are relatively low in carbohydrates and calories, and they take constant work to collect them and thus to stay alive. Early man began eating meat some 2.5 million years ago, and the fossil record shows that the human brain became remarkably bigger and more complex at this time. The incorporation of animal matter into the diet played an essential role in human evolution. The fatty acids found in meat played an important role in permitting brain growth.

The high concentration of nutrients in meat gave humans some rest from constantly gathering and eating a few vegetables. In response, the growth of the brain introduced guile and organization into societies. The meat that our ancestors ate was high in protein and low in fat. The supply was sporadic, depending upon availability and hunting skills, and a lot of energy was expended in catching it, leading to a lean and muscular habitus with a healthy frame and good nutritional status.

The presence of obesity is the basis for the development of type 2 diabetes. It used to be that children got the most aggressive, inherited type 1 diabetes. Now the majority are developing type 2 diabetes as a result of the dramatic rise of obesity in early life. Over the last twenty years, there has been a staggering 500% increase in type 2 diabetes, entirely as a result of obesity, and this will undoubtedly significantly reduce their longevity. Now, half the states in America have a prevalence of obesity of greater than 20%.

Type 2 diabetes can be prevented or completely reversed by dietary modification, weight loss, and a change in lifestyle. Remarkably, it is cured immediately in the majority of those who undergo operative gastric bypass surgery, which also improves cholesterol and blood pressure and promotes the extension of life.

Chapter 13
The Long-Term Hazards of Obesity

It has been a well-established fact that from the early thirties men with increasing weight have a progressive increase in mortality and early death. The increased mortality begins with weights just in excess of the acceptable normal range. Mortality increases with increasing weight and age thereafter, particularly in males. Excess weight gain in females is also associated with increased mortality; this begins at a somewhat older age than in men. Overweight men and women who lose weight and sustain the lost weight in a normal range can return their life expectancy to normal levels. In nonsmoking men and women, the risk of being 35 to 50% overweight, respectively, confers the same risk as smoking with a body weight within the normal range.

Obesity is an underlying risk factor in hypertension and elevated cholesterol concentrations. Other strong risk factors, as stated, are smoking, increasing age, and the male sex. Obesity also creates physical inactivity, which in turn is related to the development of heart disease. There is strong evidence that as weight increases with increasing age there is an associated elevation in blood pressure; weight loss reduces this pressure.

Kidney stone and gallstone formation are closely related to obesity and can shorten life. Gallstones probably result from the ingestion of excessive amounts of cholesterol and changes in liver function from fat infiltration, which create a further buildup of cholesterol. Gout is a problem for the obese, which damages joints and causes kidney stones. Osteoarthritis is a very common condition that occurs increasingly with increasing weight. This is a wear-and-tear process on the cartilage, which cushions and lines the joints, producing erosion and damage to the joint space, with exposure of bone on bone, producing pain and further joint destruction. It is most marked in weight-bearing joints, the hips and knees, which prevents walking and exercise, ultimately producing more weight gain and further shortening of life.

Obesity places a considerable burden on the heart and respiratory system. Lung function becomes increasingly impaired as weight increases. It further impairs exercise tolerance, and ultimately the morbidly obese patient with the combination of heart and lung impairment, together with joint disease, becomes beleaguered and totally unable to perform any exercise. Walking or climbing stairs becomes severely restricted, with some becoming ultimately bedbound.

A very common problem associated with obesity is sleep apnea. This is a condition in which levels of oxygen within the bloodstream fall, leading to sleep fragmentation, frequent wakening, and ultimately the development of heart failure. This is associated with maladies of brain function, which may occur as a result of permanent damage to the brain. The course of this condition is chronic and progressive, substantially reducing life expectancy, but it is reversible with weight loss in the early stages.

Cigarette smokers are significantly lighter than nonsmokers. Differences are often greatest in lower income groups. It is well documented that body weight increases when smokers give up their habit. While smoking is an appetite suppressant, the explanation for the weight gain that occurs when smoking is stopped may either be related to an increase in food intake or a fall in energy expenditure. Eating sweets or snacking may form substitutes for a cigarette. Smoking does slightly increase the metabolic rate by stimulating the sympathetic nervous system with nicotine. Overall, smoking is a greater hazard to life expectancy than is obesity.

The American Cancer Society has shown an association between obesity and an increased risk of cancer of the colon, rectum, and prostate. With increasing weight, women show a progressive increase in the risk of cancer of the breast, uterus, and cervix.

Deep vein thrombosis and pulmonary embolisms are a common cause of sudden death, more common in obese patients. Infectious diseases leading to septicemia and multiple organ failure and death are also more common in the obese.

Why do people become obese? The basic answer is because in the long term they ingest calories far in excess of their needs. It has been shown that the obese inherit a lower metabolic rate than normal individuals, and it is hereditary, but as they gain weight, the metabolic rate increases to provide energy for the maintenance of their excess weight.

Obesity now often begins early in life. There has been a threefold increase in the incidence of obesity in three and four-year-old children in the last twenty years. During this time, there has been no change in birth weight and no change in the gene pool. Thus, obesity in children is acquired, relating principally to lifestyle, and tends to persist throughout life. Factors that contribute to this are: the increased consumption of fast food and high calorie drinks, reduced physical activity brought on by fixed television viewing, food advertising, and less breastfeeding. These factors are strongly influenced by parents.

We should never underestimate the power of advertising. Advertising is a powerful factor in the vicious equation that has developed concerning the effect of lifestyle on longevity. Food marketers target children and adults to influence their food choices and eating behavior. So lucrative is this business that one large company contracts to provide free computers and televisions to schools in exchange for compelling the children to view two minutes of commercial messages each day. Food advertising makes up a large proportion of this viewing time, as it does on mainline television. This perhaps reflects upon the way in which the nation's schools are funded. In relative terms, education has become increasingly poorly financed, which could have long-term consequences later in life. Furthermore, the effects of the advertising campaigns are surreptitious and difficult to evaluate. We are all immersed in the sea of advertising to a greater degree than we are aware. If advertising was not so powerful and influential, companies would not invest the billions of dollars that go into the industry. Observation of the plethora of advertising on television, in the press, on the Internet, and on our streets only goes to emphasize its relevance and effect on all of our lives.

Our experience gained in passing through the educational system provides a foundation for subsequent life experiences that affect longevity, and there are significant differences in life expectancy that relate to educational achievements and subsequent careers. In the past decade, in some school districts, fast food companies took over food service operations. Under these circumstances, the fast food company eliminates the burden to the school of providing meals that children will eat. The question of appropriate nutrition, physical activity, and weight management never entered the equation. These meal services are often supplemented by vending machines, which provide an endless supply of sugar that is accessible throughout the day.

Over a period of twenty years, soda sales to school distributors increased by 1100%. Each can of Coke contains the equivalent of ten teaspoons of sugar. One large soda can supply one half of the total daily caloric intake required by a teenager, and the average child consumes more than one can of soda per day. There is a direct correlation between soda consumption and obesity in childhood. Another factor in present-day schooling has been the reduction in physical education and exercise. Soda consumption combined with an increasing lack of exercise is a potent combination in the production of obesity, which remains long term and reduces longevity.

Social factors driving obesity in childhood have been generated by, and are equally present, in adults. Adults now walk less, drive more cars, use more public transport, and eat in more restaurants than ever before. There are more elevators, escalators, conveyor belts, automated industries, televisions, computers, robots, and couches. Conversely, there are more gymnasiums, sales of exercise equipment, jogging tracks, and other sports facilities. The latter, however, are only used by a small preselected cross section of the community, but because of the physical encumbrance and embarrassment produced by their obesity, these people tend not to use these aids.

The exact mechanism by which man controls his energy intake to maintain a steady weight is not fully understood. A "set point" seems to exist, which in practical terms is a buffer zone around which most people keep their weight approximately constant.

Factors affecting the set point are: satiety, a feeling of adequate food intake, distention of the stomach, and the effects of stimulating nerve fibers between the stomach and the brain. In trying to maintain the set point, the body intrinsically attempts to control its caloric intake. Increased intake stimulates energy and activity, whereas decreased intake tends to reduce physical activity through an expression of tiredness or the induction of a restful state. It is possible for the body to reset the set-point in an upward direction so that prolonged and continuous excess food intake ultimately produces an elevation of the set point to an increased weight. Conversely, the body's defense of the set-point has been used to explain why the maintenance of medically induced weight loss has been so poor and is, in the long term, for most people, a failure.

Energy conservation is a factor that influences short-term weight stability. So often one hears people complain that they have virtually starved for a few days and not lost any weight. This is due to the functional aspect of the set-point, when in this conservation mode the body reduces energy output by reducing the metabolic rate to compensate for the sudden shut off of food intake. This is probably not only confined to the metabolic rate but also to energy usage by the body for exercise and day-to-day activities. Such conservation is related to the maintenance of the set-point.

Many who suffer from obesity feel that their underlying problem is hormonal or glandular and that the thyroid gland, in particular, is the source of the problem. There is no evidence that obese patients have different thyroid hormone responses to changes in energy than normal non-obese individuals. Underactivity of the thyroid gland, a condition called myxedema, will predispose to obesity just as the over activity, which is called thyrotoxicosis, is associated with weight loss and increased sympathetic activity. It is for this reason that many have attempted to use thyroid hormones to stimulate metabolism and produce weight loss. Increased levels of thyroid hormones do increase the patient's metabolic rate but may produce undesirable and potentially dangerous complications such as cardiac rhythm disturbances, which may lead to cardiac failure, atrial fibrillation, stroke, and even sudden death. Anxiety, tremors, sweating, and palpitations are other side effects of the use of thyroid hormones. Where thyroxine has been used in the treatment of obesity, the results have been unimpressive.

Excessive production of steroids by the adrenal gland, Cushing's syndrome, may produce obesity, but the condition is distinctly uncommon and rarely contributes to the problem of the underlying weight gain in the obese patient. Many subjects are taking prescription steroids for a variety of conditions, most commonly rheumatological conditions. These are antiinflammatory agents, but they produce a number of side effects in addition to obesity, chiefly hypertension, stroke, osteoporosis, and peptic ulceration. They produce an alteration of body habitus with a dysmorphic appearance, a buffalo hump and thick neck, a distended abdomen, and marked muscle loss and weakness in the limbs.

In this body-conscious country, bodybuilding has become increasingly popular. The taking of androgenic steroids, male sex hormones, will add to muscle mass and produce a redistribution of muscle, with broad shoulders, large pectorals, a six-pack in the abdomen, and muscular quadriceps in the legs. This may help the weightlifter, but there is no evidence that it prolongs life, and it probably predisposes to hypertension, stroke, and coronary artery disease.

Sex hormones influence the accumulation and distribution of fat. Females tend to have a higher percentage of body fat than males, and most morbidly obese people are female. The distribution of fat is also different between the sexes, which is hormonally related. Males deposit fat on their central abdomens and become potbellied. Females concentrate the fat on their lower abdomen, pelvis, and thighs. Males have been described as being "apple-shaped" and females as "pear-shaped."

Growth hormone has been advocated for use in weight loss programs and has also been used in an attempt to preserve male strength and promote longevity. The use of growth hormone does alter body habitus by redistributing fat and promoting muscle growth, which it undoubtedly achieves. Demand for it is great, particularly from athletes such as football and baseball players, but there is no evidence that it prolongs life.

In recent years, there has been much interest in gut hormones, which, with variable interdependence, have been promoted to reduce food intake and produce weight loss. These hormones affect the secretion of acid by the stomach and of pancreatic juice. There is no hard scientific evidence that any of these hormones play a significant role in controlling obesity. These hormones are leptin, resistin, neuropeptide Y, C-75, and grehlin. There have been several recent important studies and observations that may assist in our understanding of the cause and treatment of obesity, but the interaction of these hormones is complex and further research is required to elucidate the situation.

Fat storage evolved over millions of years as a primary mechanism for coping with periods of famine, as an inferior method to that evolved by animals in hibernation. For most of the evolutionary pathway, the major problem has been getting enough food to eat in order to survive the winter, rather than avoiding obesity. When calorie intake exceeds expenditure, fat cells swell to as much as six times their minimum size, and they begin to multiply. In the average adult, there are forty billion fat cells, which can increase up to one hundred billion. Losing weight causes fat cells to shrink in size and become less metabolically active, but their number, once present, goes down only very slowly, if at all.

The process of inflammation can be a major killer. Fat cells promote inflammation, which can spread throughout the body. Even small amounts of excess fat can produce a mounting immune response, which can give rise to multiple organ failure, a highly fatal situation. This is because the body regards the storage of excess fat cells as an invading organism and attempts to reject it by mounting an inflammatory response, as if it were dealing with an infective organism. Inflammation is now viewed as a key mechanism in producing heart disease, probably being more important than cholesterol levels, per se. The coronary arteries are undoubtedly narrowed by cholesterol, but a big problem appears to be that an inflamed plaque can break open, produce a clot and occlude the vessel, a process known as coronary thrombosis.

In the case of the coronary arteries, blockage leads to death of the cardiac muscle, which is fed by these vessels. Compounds secreted by fat cells contribute to vascular inflammation, and they inhibit nitric oxide, a chemical that helps relax blood vessels and lowers blood pressure. Fat cells also secrete estrogen, which is linked to certain types of cancer. Researchers now suspect that the origin of diabetes lies, at least partly, in the biochemistry of fat, in particular into compounds made by fat cells. These are called resistin and tumor necrosis factor. Resistin promotes the conversion of fatty acids into glucose by the liver, a process that is useful during starvation, but a potential hazard for the obese patient. The amount of resistin that the body produces increases with the amount of fat stored. Tumor necrosis factor, a naturally occurring substance, promotes insulin resistance.

In different parts of the body, fat cells behave differently and are of different types. Fat carried in the hips and thighs is considered comparatively benign, whereas that which accumulates around organs in the abdomen, described as brown fat, is more harmful. The latter is more metabolically active and produces more inflammation and clot-promoting compounds than does fat distributed around the periphery of the body. Fortunately, visceral brown fat is the first to disappear in response to exercise and diet. The actual distribution of body fat is genetically determined, but the amount of fat stored relates directly to excess intake over output.

"It's my genes" is a common cry of people apologizing for their obesity but unable to do anything about it. Obesity genes have been identified, but their role is ill-defined and unlikely to be major. Overall balance between energy intake and expenditure is a fine one, and only small daily deviations, if continued in the long term, can have a large effect upon weight. A 1% excess of intake over energy expenditure stored as fat would produce a weight gain of two pounds in a year, fifty pounds in twenty years. Achieving this accurate balance depends upon a complex interaction of hormones, activity, temperature exposure, and other factors. The gut hormones referred to above have an extremely complex relationship with each other, one which is not yet understood. All of them act in concert to maintain the set point. Genetic variations can lead some people to eat more, and eating habits start in the family and are maintained in the long term, so obesity is by and large a behavioral problem without underlying genetic, psychiatric, or hormonally detectable abnormalities.

Being obese can raise the risk of dying early by 50%. Even being slightly overweight raises the incidence of illnesses like type 2 diabetes and arthritis. A recent survey of 2.8 million people concluded that overweight individuals are at a heightened risk of developing ten of twelve severe conditions. These include stroke, heart failure, angina, sleep apnea, and renal failure.

People were divided into five groups based on their body mass index. The groups had BMIs of less than 25, 25 to 29, 30 to 35, 35 to 39, or over 40. Being just slightly overweight doubles the incidence of type 2 diabetes, raises the risk of arthritis by 33%, asthma by 28%, and high blood pressure by 50%. They also had a 70% higher risk of heart failure and 60% for renal failure.

Those with a BMI of over 40 had a risk of type 2 diabetes more than twelve times that of a normal weight person, and the risk of sleep apnea was twenty-two times higher. Men were more likely to develop these complications than women. These findings have serious implications for public health. Being overweight creates insulin resistance. The obesity epidemic is reaching a highly alarming situation, which puts an enormous strain on the cost of healthcare; type 2 diabetes sufferers account for 11% of the total bills for prescription drugs. People must pay more attention to their own and their children's diet and exercise.

Chapter 14
The Psychology of the Obese State

Although underlying psychiatric disorders can rarely be identified as being causative for obesity, psychiatric problems are commonly associated with the obese state once it has developed. It is hardly surprising that the morbidly obese individual who cannot climb a flight of stairs, run, sit in a conventional seat, get on a bus or an aircraft, or wear attractive clothes, would have low self-esteem. Low self-esteem leads to social isolation, which, in terms of longevity, is not good. Many obese people will not go out of the house in daylight hours because they are so self-conscious. Social isolation leads to depression, and food provides solace to the depressed. Associated physical disorders such as sleep apnea, diabetes, hypertension, and vascular disease can lead to adverse mental changes.

It has been said that the massively increased prevalence of obesity in recent years cannot be attributed to either a change in genetics or recognizable psychiatric disorders. It is rather clearly behavioral, cultural, a submission to extrinsic pressures such as food advertisements, and a consequence of an acquired aberration of the role and value of nutrients. Such behavioral influences may have led more people to "live to eat" rather than "eat to live". This would suggest addictive behavior, of which there may clearly be a component. Addiction to food is ostensibly more of a problem than addiction to alcohol or drugs because, difficult as the latter are to manage, the patient may be excluded from access to alcohol, while food is a necessity. Not only is food essential—we are what we eat—its accurate balance, as a fundamental need provider, may be extremely difficult to control once the regular homeostatic control mechanisms fall away.

The homeostatic mechanisms that regulate eating behavior throughout the animal kingdom are becoming grossly distorted in man for the first time in thousands of years. Throughout history, man has suffered more from the ravages of starvation than from a plethora of food, but gluttony and obesity existed with other excesses in the period of affluence during the Roman era. Although gross effects of malnutrition and the extremes of starvation in central Africa and other countries are depicted by the media, we may have entered an era where more die from an excess than a shortage of food.

Numerous biological and psychological influences may modify eating behavior. Dietary composition, per se, is not an exact determinant of body makeup. As both protein and carbohydrate can be efficiently converted into fat, there is no evidence that changing the relative proportions of protein, carbohydrate, and fat in the diet without reducing overall caloric intake will promote weight loss.

The fact that psychological factors are important in governing caloric intake is clear when we look at studies that attempt to eliminate these factors. A study was carried out in which preweighed bottles of milk were delivered to the houses of thirtyseven babies. The bottles were then collected for reweighing for the determination of food intake. By varying the dilution of the milk, different energy densities of which the mothers were unaware of were given at different times. The babies fed with halfstrength milk increased their volume intake by 80%, but not 100%. This would suggest that appetite may be related in part to volume intake rather than energy intake. A study like this would not be possible later in life, but it suggested drinking lots of water is good.

Studies in older malnourished children in Jamaica, however, demonstrated the development of a voracious appetite after longterm food deprivation. This might be an explanation for the often observed rapid weight gain that follows a period of dieting. Psychological factors do impose a considerable influence on dietary intake, which is also influenced by the color, texture, smell, taste, and the energy content of food. Studies have shown that an individual's selection of food reflects a response to food availability and palatability, rather than energy content, hence the effect of fast foods in producing weight gain. These factors are social as well as psychological. The situation is complex, in that animals may vary their intake and accordingly obtain sufficient amounts of essential minerals and vitamins when food concentrations of these are low. If such instincts ever existed in man, they have now probably been lost.

Societies across the world have developed an antagonistic attitude towards obesity. Obese children tend to be looked down upon, even disliked, cajoled, and bullied. Their obese state from a very young age is associated with shame, as they are thought to be self-indulgent and lacking in willpower. They are regarded as being responsible for their own condition, whereas disabled children receive sympathy and support, but the situation is very complex. Obese patients tend to beget or create obese children. The availability and palatability of food influences intake. Highcalorie value of food tends to equate with palatability, and foods high in sugar content are more accessible by being cheaper. Social and family pressures can lead to overeating, as it is often regarded as a sign of appreciation to eat all of the food presented. Important life events such as birthdays, successes, marriages, and even funerals are celebrated by feasts.

Such practices are not new. The Romans derived great pleasure from eating, and often overeating, in a gluttonous fashion. "Ear ticklers" existed in Roman times, people who were skilled at rubbing the area behind the ears of those who had overeaten, inducing vomiting and thereby enabling the partygoer to begin eating again. The mechanism of this procedure was that the vagus nerve supplies not only the stomach but also extends to branches behind the ear. Stimulation of the ear activates the vagus nerve, producing contractions of the stomach that induce vomiting.

Throughout life, the eating of food becomes an important ritual. We all like good foods, a variety of foods, and we not only socialize around the table, we hold business meetings as well. If indeed food becomes an addiction, which is the case in some morbidly obese individuals, then it is one with which the addicted must constantly contend, as food is not only essential, it is around as always. Diets eaten in different countries vary widely, but most nations have, over the centuries, developed diets that, though widely differing in their content, maintain the body in good functional health without any marked nutritional deficiencies. Recently, studies have shown that Puerto Rican women living in the continental United States increase weight the longer they have spent there and the better their English. This is persuasive evidence that social factors rather than genetic ones are important.

Though perhaps difficult to accurately categorize the psychological effects, factors that pertain to the obese state are significant and considerable. The higher the BMI, the greater is the incidence of depression. A number of factors contribute to the development of psychological problems that culminate in chronic depression, a harbinger of early suicide. Discrimination leads to low self-worth and a reduced quality of life. Family and sexual relationships suffer, and problems frequently arise in the workplace, making employment difficult and disadvantaged. Over two-thirds of obese patients report abuse, physical in 34%, sexual in 12%, and psychological in 64%. One-third of obese patients report a family history of alcoholism. Conversely, alcoholism is rare in the morbidly obese subject.

Body image can greatly affect lifestyle. Those abused in childhood may use their obese state as a protection against attracting men. Despite their desire to lose weight, they may get more and more anxious as they lose some weight and become shapelier, and thus attractive. Another person who equates food with love, or weight with power and affluence, will experience much inner conflict about changing their lifestyle when losing weight.

To be successful, all psychotherapists must address emotional dysregulation, impulsive behavior, and cognitive or perceptual distortions. Group and individual therapy, particularly cognitive behavioral therapy, can highlight rationalizations, reframe negative patterns of thinking, and provide a more realistic manner of self-assessment. A recognition of one's own mental functioning and how one solves problems is essential to those attitudes from the past that may sabotage dieting efforts.

Early in the twentieth century, when tuberculosis and other infectious diseases were still rampant, to be thin was often perceived as a sign of sickness, poverty, or neglect. The prize of families was to have plump, "healthy" children. The plump female was womanly and beautiful; look at the art of those days. The plump male, watch chain stretched across his belly, looked prosperous. People paid little or no attention to the calorie content of what they ate.

When World War II brought rationing, meat and butter became luxury items. Gas was rationed, people walked, yet most middle-aged adults in the US were overweight, and few exercised for health. There were few gymnasiums. Most women over thirty would lose their figure and wear a tight-fitting girdle. Men padded their shoulders and wore double-breasted suits to hide middle-aged bellies; it was thought to be natural and nothing was done about it. This was the time when heart attacks and strokes began to mushroom.

After the war, television produced a big change in lifestyle and led to a major change in eating habits, none for the better. The "TV dinner" became prominent, and everyone gathered around the new center in the home, eating the fast foods they saw advertised on the screen. Television's advertising potential became huge and was quickly realized and exploited by the food industry. Advertising showed America the face it wanted to see: big, affluent, carefree, untouched by war or want. Things became oversized, cars sported huge fins and contained three-seater cross benches that were capacious with room for all. In the new supermarkets, myriad food packages promised more for your money, and restaurants served larger portions. Consequently, Americans learned to overeat and enjoyed it, but they paid the price in health terms.

Chapter 15
Nutritional Requirements

Nutritional requirements vary with age, sex, and body size and can be influenced by drugs, hormones, and disease states. Carbohydrates provide approximately half the human energy requirement. They are ingested either as simple sugars or more complex carbohydrates. Certain tissues such as the brain, blood cells, and kidneys have an essential requirement for glucose.

Lipids, as well as being a source of energy, play an important role in the structure and function of cells. Proteins make up 20% of the lean body mass as muscle. Proteins exist in the form of enzymes, which are required to enable chemical reactions to be carried out inside the body. Another important role of proteins is to provide a source of essential amino acids. These are the amino acids that are required for normal body function and cannot be produced by the body. Dietary proteins contain these essential amino acids in varying concentrations.

Many of the normal chemical processes essential for life require vitamins. Deficiencies of these vitamins cause welldefined diseases. A total of thirteen vitamins have been identified as being essential in human nutrition. Five of these are fat-soluble and eight are water-soluble. The fat-soluble vitamins are A, D, E and K. Vitamins A, C, and E, together with the mineral selenium, are antioxidants, important in the breakdown of free radical oxidation products. One vitamin deficiency well known to the public is scurvy, which historically used to be common on long sea voyages. Scurvy, which presents with bleeding from the gums, is due to a deficiency of vitamin C, or ascorbic acid. On long transatlantic sea voyages, sailors became deficient in vitamin C and developed a full-blown syndrome of scurvy, which ultimately became preventable and treatable by the provision of limes to sailors embarking on long voyages, hence the name for British sailors: "limeys."

In addition to vitamins, there are nineteen minerals and trace minerals that are all essential to humans and may be grouped into four categories based on their function. Calcium, phosphorous, magnesium, and zinc are structural components of bone. A second group—sodium, potassium, and chloride—function as major charged ions within the cellular mechanism. Trace minerals, which are necessary for normal health, include iron, zinc, copper, selenium, manganese, molybdenum, cobalt, iodine, and chromium.

Minerals are necessary to prevent disease states, and the intake of minerals can be low even in the obese state, but particularly so following surgery for morbid obesity. Malabsorption, the consequence of a number of diseases, like Crohn's disease, and the effects of some drugs can alter mineral balances. Farmers working on land deficient in certain minerals such as iron will put blocks of the deficient mineral in their fields, which animals such as sheep and cows instinctively come down and lick to overcome their deficiency.

Calcium is the most abundant mineral in the body and plays a vital role in muscular and cardiac activity. It is also involved in the coagulation of the blood and the handling of certain hormones. High levels of calcium can cause kidney stones; low levels cause brittle bones, which are prone to spontaneous fractures. Low levels of calcium may also be associated with low levels of albumin and magnesium. Magnesium is an essential important mineral within cells and is involved in many chemical reactions. A common manifestation of zinc deficiency is hair loss. Low levels of iron due to either inadequate ingestion or bleeding produces anemia, which can be profound.

CHAPTER 16
MAINTAINING A HEALTHY WEIGHT

Maintaining a healthy weight adds to longevity and enables adequate exercise. People whose weight is in the normal range have a reduced incidence of all the major killers. It has been estimated that, at any one time, two-thirds of women and one-third of men are trying to lose weight. Over one-third of the population are regular users of one or more slimming products, which are widely and persistently advertised, particularly on television. Overall, most attempted slimming is self-administered and selfcontrolled without supervision. There are no authoritative guidelines for health education of the general public regarding the optimal type of diet.

A large number of commercial diets are available for weightloss programs. Women's magazines, and even specialist magazines, that are totally devoted to the subject exist in large numbers. Industry has become very calorie conscious, listing dietary contents and calories on most packages. Low-calorie breads and zero-calorie drinks are now prominently displayed on supermarket shelves. Numerous slimming items are available, and specialized shops and Internet companies exist. Short-term weight loss can be achieved, but there is little scientific evidence that any of these products achieve long-term weight loss.

Organizations and magazines run self-help groups. These magazines give substantive advice on slimming, but often project incorrect nutritional principles. They frequently advocate crash diets—"lose 12 pounds in the first week"—which almost invariably lead to rebound weight gain, or they focus on specific foodstuffs that may be inappropriate for a long-term strategy in achieving weight loss.

Historically, diets have focused on reduced fat intake. For almost a century, emphasis has been placed, by the medical profession, on reducing the intake of animal fat in dairy products. Fat contains nine calories per gram, as opposed to four calories for carbohydrates and protein, but fat is not so easily eaten in large amounts as are carbohydrates, and carbohydrate excesses are converted into fat.

Successful weight reduction depends on a number of factors. The most important is to control calorie intake in the long term. This involves staying approximately on a particular dietary scheme. Individuals' energy requirements vary considerably, so the results achieved by specific diets can be different.

On most calorie-counting diets, the subject is allowed to eat any foods that cumulatively provide a given energy intake. Although there is freedom of choice, there are many disadvantages. Food needs to be weighed precisely, and energy intake is counted from this. Commonly, people will state that these diets fail, when in reality it is unlikely that the patient is adhering to the diet. A slight variation on this theme is the "set diet," in which a diet sheet provides the week's menu for three meals per day. These menus offer a variety, and alternatives are frequently given. Eating an additional 1% would amount to an extra ten thousand calories per year; that is just over a can of cola per day and will cause a gain of two pounds per year, equivalent to walking a hundred miles.

With low-fat diets, the individual is provided with a list of foods that are high in fat that must be avoided or severely restricted. These diets often originated specifically to reduce cholesterol levels and thereby reduce the risk of heart disease. Carbohydrates are not usually specifically restricted with these diets, which usually fail.

Currently, the most popular and effective diets are those that are low in carbohydrates, and these diets go back a long way. Banting, who discovered insulin over a century ago, devised lowcarbohydrate diets for treating diabetes. They are now used as a major strategy for weight loss and increased longevity. The most widely used are the Atkins diet, Sugar Busters, and the South Beach diet.

The Atkins diet, as claimed by the late author, is an easy-to-stay-with regime that combines nutrition and vital nutrient supplements into a unique, not only weight-reducing, but also age-defying program.

Atkins claimed that his diet adds many years to life, boosts immune defenses, enhances brain function and memory, reduces the risk of cardiovascular disease, permits weight loss without calorie restriction, and combats adult-onset diabetes. Atkins promulgated this diet against strong opposition from august bodies such as the American Cardiological Society.

The Atkins diet involves a radical reduction of intake of carbohydrates. Those carbohydrates that are allowed are complex and unrefined, basically starchy foods including whole grains and lentils. Table sugar, sweets, cakes, cookies, and sodas are banned. These latter foods have a very high glycemic index that sends insulin levels soaring. Simple carbohydrates should be no more than about 3% of the total diet. Pasta, bread, white rice, baked goods, and candy are forbidden.

Simple sugars are banned because they are rapidly digested and bump up the blood sugar, producing a rapid outpouring of large amounts of insulin from the pancreas. This causes the glucose level to fall and creates a craving for more carbohydrates. As insulin resistance develops, the excess sugar accumulates in the blood, producing diabetes. This situation also leads to obesity, as the excess sugar is ultimately converted into fat. Atkins conceded that trans fats are the dietary link to elevated cholesterol and heart disease. Trans fats lower the good HDL-cholesterol and raise the bad LDL-cholesterol and lipoproteins. Trans fats also reduce responsiveness to insulin and block the uptake of essential fatty acids. Atkins advocated taking a wide variety of foods that will supply an array of vital nutrients and phytochemicals and avoid any potential for addiction to a particular foodstuff. As its first objective, the Atkins diet stabilizes blood sugar by eliminating simple sugars and sugar-containing foods and replacing them with either complex carbohydrates or non-carbohydrates.

The diet is based on a much higher than normal fat and protein content. A second objective is to create a diet that is low in foods that create oxygen-free radicals and high in antioxidants that fight them. To increase antioxidant capacity, the diet is high in fresh vegetables and low-sugar fruits such as berries.

An advantage of the diet is that the patient does not have to count calories or even excessively restrict portion size. Steak and fish may be eaten with free access to fresh vegetables. Brown rice and genuine whole-grain bread are allowed. Some cheeses are permitted without restriction, but yogurts, which are high in lactose, a simple sugar, should be minimized. Bran, nuts, and seeds are permitted. Butter is preferred to margarine, as the latter is high in trans fats. Fat intake also helps stabilize blood sugar levels.

The best oils are olive oil, almond, and avocado. These oils are excellent sources of omega-3 and omega-6 essential fatty acids.

Replacement of simple carbohydrates with high-quality complex carbohydrates, which are starches, is advocated. Complex carbohydrates are more likely to keep the blood sugar steady when they are combined with protein and fat. Green vegetables can be eaten freely, including salad greens, broccoli, kale, Brussels sprouts, and green beans. Carrots, beets, peas, and winter squash are higher in carbohydrates, though they are also high in antioxidants. Potatoes are not encouraged; if taken, they should be eaten with skins. Fruits should only be taken in moderation. They are rich in vitamins and minerals, but they contain significant amounts of simple carbohydrates. Fruit juices and canned fruits should be avoided; they have no nutritional value and are loaded with sugar.

The Atkins diet emphasizes the importance of drinking large amounts of fluid, but not soda. Teas and coffee are allowed; alcoholic beverages may be taken in moderation. Several studies have shown that a glass of red wine has a beneficial effect on the heart and blood vessels, but this is controversial. As has been stated, there is a lot of uncertainty relating to alcohol intake, and it is wisest to drink moderate amounts of dry wine or straight liquor with a sugarless mixture such as zero-calorie soda. Beer and dessert wines should be avoided. The controversies surrounding the drinking of alcohol have yet to be resolved. Alcohol does, however, increase HDL, good cholesterol, and decreases platelet stickiness and their aggregation, which promote thrombosis. These actions tend to reduce the development of arteriosclerosis and are most likely to be achieved when red wine, rather than any other form of alcohol, is ingested. A number of studies have shown that the number of deaths from cancer, heart disease, strokes, and accidents are cumulatively reduced in people who take one or two alcoholic beverages per day, but not more than three. Those who drink more than three run a higher relative risk of death from all causes, and with increasing the amount further, there is a significant risk of death from cirrhosis of the liver and gastrointestinal bleeding.

With regard to the amount of food taken, Atkins recommended eating until comfortable. Food that is free of carbohydrates satisfies the appetite more rapidly. Overeating becomes almost impossible. It is recommended to take a highprotein breakfast and three full meals per day. Vegetables have considerably more antioxidants per carbohydrate grams than fruit and are a valuable dietary choice. The best choice among the fruits are berries of any kind. A cup of blueberries contains only forty calories. Avocados are excellent sources of monounsaturated fats.

There has been much discussion recently about the importance of carotenoids. It has been claimed that the carotenoid lycopene may prevent cancer, particularly cancer of the prostate. This chemical has now been added to many over-the-counter multivitamin preparations. Sources of these are dark green leafy vegetables and orange colored foods such as carrots and tomatoes.

Without carbohydrates, the body does not burn fat efficiently and produces compounds called ketones, which accumulate in the blood and are toxic. These cause nausea, headache, fatigue, and constipation and put a strain on the kidneys. Whether this diet increases the risk of heart disease, vascular disease, and even cancer remains controversial, but no scientific evidence of this exists, and the diet is associated with reduced levels of serum cholesterol. Unfortunately, Atkins himself died suddenly of a heart attack while jogging.

A low-carbohydrate diet that is very widely used is the Sugar Busters diet, which emphasizes that sugar is toxic. It is stressed that the overproduction of insulin causes the body to store excess energy as fat. Insulin further inhibits the mobilization of previously stored fat, and insulin signals the liver to make cholesterol. The Sugar Busters diet, which is most widely advertised, prohibits carbohydrates that cause an intense insulin secretion; these are refined sugars. Foods that must be eliminated from this diet are potatoes, corn, white rice, bread from refined flour, beets, carrots, granulated sugar, corn syrup, molasses, honey, colas, and beer.

Red wine, which is regarded as the best and safest source of alcohol, is allowed with the Sugar Busters diet. Populations in countries with a higher relative consumption of red wine compared to other spirits experience a lower incidence of cardiovascular disease. Alcohol, however, is high in calories. With the Sugar Busters diet, exercise is endorsed as a definite plus. Modulating insulin is the key to this diet. Successfully controlling insulin allows the patient to unlock improved performance through health and nutrition. To control insulin secretion, it is fundamental that the intake of sugar is reduced and that refined carbohydrates are cut down to a minimum. Avoiding refined carbohydrates results in lower average insulin levels in the blood for prolonged periods of time. This has a remarkably beneficial effect on reducing fat synthesis and storage, as well as mitigating other adverse influences that insulin has on the cardiovascular system. Along with the Atkins philosophy, here it is also emphasized that refined carbohydrates are very rapidly absorbed, resulting in the secretion of large amounts of insulin that promotes fat deposition. Unrefined carbohydrates, however, require more digestive breakdown before absorption. The slower absorption modulates insulin secretion and results in less fat synthesis and storage and consequently less weight gain.

The Sugar Busters diet sensibly does not ban all carbohydrates. There is a particular emphasis on completely avoiding refined sugars, and this works. Many diets advocate eliminating almost all fat and meat, especially red meat. Some fat in the diet is necessary for the completion of metabolic operations within the body. Most of the excess fat is due to the conversion of ingested carbohydrates to fat. Proponents of the Sugar Busters diet place great emphasis on the eating of meat, which may not be its strong point. They state that ingested protein stimulates production of the hormone glucagon as well as providing building blocks for the body. Glucagon promotes the breakdown of stored fat and helps counteract the effects of high insulin levels on the cardiovascular system.

The proponents of the Sugar Busters diet place emphasis on eating patterns or habits. Multiple meals place less stimulus on insulin secretion by causing the body to enter a conservation mode. This tends to increase fat storage, possibly peripherally, associated with the ability, which some mammals have, to hibernate. It is recommended that we should eat three meals a day to prevent the conservation mode from developing.

Both the Atkins and the Sugar Busters diets do not count calories, which tends to be very inaccurate. It is also not necessary to count sugar grams, fat grams, or protein grams. Overall portion size is not restricted, provided that it consists of high-fiber carbohydrates, lean meats, and unsaturated fats. Unlike the Atkins diet, Sugar Busters expresses concern about eating too much fat, especially saturated fats. In the Sugar Busters diet, portions of food should fit on the bottom of the plate; second and third helpings are discouraged. It is beneficial to consume calories early in the day and eating a large meal at night is considered bad. Ingested cholesterol leads to deposition in the arterial system and ultimately to thrombosis. Between meal snacks are discouraged. Fruits are less good than vegetables but contain fructose, which has approximately one-third of the insulin secretion created by glucose. Fruits should be eaten whole, and fruit juices are discouraged.

Both of these diets recommend a large sugar-free liquid intake, particularly before meals. Tea and coffee are discouraged, but other scientific studies have recommended them in moderation. It is recommended that six to eight glasses of water should be consumed per day, which tends to curb appetite. Breakfast cereals are laced with sugar and are discouraged. Wheat bread, which is whole grain, should replace white bread.

As well as reducing insulin secretion, the Sugar Busters diet stimulates the production of glucagon, thus reducing body fat and cholesterol and the health problems associated with them. It is important that the major protein source should be lean white meat and fish. These should be grilled, baked, or broiled, but not fried. Egg consumption is controversial. The egg yolk contains 185 mg of cholesterol. Nuts and avocados are a healthy source of fats. Sugar Busters claims to be creating a new nutritional lifestyle. It is logical, well-founded, practical, and reasonable, being not too difficult to follow. Unlike the Atkins diet, Sugar Busters aims at removing unnecessary fat, especially saturated fat, from the diet and concentrating on the ingestion of lean and trimmed meats. Refined carbohydrates are again banned. Sugar Busters forms a sensible long-term guide to lifestyle and can be recommended.

The South Beach diet claims to be neither low-carb nor low-fat. The aim is to teach reliance on the right carbohydrates and the right fats. As a weight reducing diet, it is claimed that between eight and thirteen pounds can be lost in the first two weeks. Free access is allowed to vegetables, chicken, turkey, fish, and shellfish. Acceptable fats are eggs, cheese, nuts, and olive oil; even snacks are permitted. Bread, rice, potatoes, pasta, and baked goods are completely prohibited, as is fruit. Cakes, cookies, ice cream, and sugar are also banned. Alcohol, in moderation, is allowed, of which red wine is again thought best. It is claimed that the diet produces a loss of abdominal fat, which is usually the most difficult area of fat to reduce. The initial program can be relaxed after a few weeks, but the underlying principles should still be adhered to. The diet is safe, relatively simple, and in some ways similar to Sugar Busters. These two diets form excellent guidelines for one's long-term healthy eating strategy, without being too restrictive or intolerable.

It is of interest that the South Beach diet was devised by Arthur Agatston, a cardiologist who had grown disillusioned with the low-fat, high-carbohydrate diet that had for many years been recommended by the American Heart Association. As a consequence, he introduced the South Beach diet in the mid-1990s. Focus was placed on the prevention of the myriad heart and vascular problems that stem from obesity. While placing emphasis on the beneficial effects on the cardiovascular system, Dr Agatston also focused on the importance and beneficial effects of losing weight from a cosmetic standpoint, which is a strong motivating factor for continuing with the diet. The psychological lift that comes from an improved appearance benefits the entire person and keeps many a patient from backsliding. The end result is to improve general and cardiovascular health, with a better, more active, and positive body habitus and attitude. To make up for the radical cut in carbohydrates, people ate more protein and fat, and the diets were for some hard to adhere to; this particularly applied to the Atkins diet. The South Beach diet is probably the easiest to stay with in the long term, but the Sugar Busters diet is probably more effective, if the focus is primarily on weight reduction.

An important principle of the South Beach diet is to permit good carbohydrates, vegetables, whole grains and some fruits to be taken while excluding the highly processed bad carbohydrates. By permitting the taking of lean beef, pork, veal and lamb it is easier to stay on this diet then on the more radical Sugar Busters.

The South Beach diet allows egg yolks, which contain a lot of vitamin E and good, as well as bad cholesterol, but with about 185 mg of cholesterol in an egg, the number taken per week should be reduced, perhaps reasonably to three. Chicken, turkey, fish—especially salmon, tuna and mackerel—are recommended, along with nuts, low-fat cheeses, and yogurt. Olive oil, canola oil, and peanut oil are considered good, containing healthy fats. One of Agatston's criticisms of the Atkins diet is that the extreme limitation of carbohydrates leads to the breakdown of fats, producing ketosis. To otherwise relatively healthy overweight individuals, this is probably not harmful and may be associated with a decrease in blood volume and some dehydration, which could affect kidney function, causing permanent renal damage in the long term.

The major concern that has always surrounded the Atkins diet, theoretically, is that following a meal of saturated fats, there is dysfunction in the arteries, which results in deposits on the arterial wall linings of cholesterol plaques, thus the predisposition to thrombosis. The question remains unresolved, but it is real, and these adverse effects do not occur when unsaturated fats are consumed.

In a randomized controlled clinical trial involving fasting overweight volunteers, the South Beach diet was compared with the American Heart Association program. After twelve weeks, five patients on the AHA program had given up, compared with just one on the South Beach diet. South Beach dieters experienced a mean weight loss of 13.6 pounds, almost double the 7.5 pounds lost by the AHA group. Those on the South Beach diet also showed a greater decrease in waist-to-hip ratio, suggesting a true decrease in cardiac risk. Cholesterol levels for those on the South Beach diet dramatically decreased, and the good-to-bad cholesterol ratio improved more than in those of the Heart Association group. It is clear that much of the insulin resistance syndrome disappears after two weeks on the South Beach diet. The cravings for sugars virtually disappeared.

A little olive oil will enhance the process of slowing down the absorption of carbohydrates. Also, taking a spoonful of Metamucil in a glass of water before a meal can have a similar benefit. Nonsoluble fiber mixed with the food has the effect of slowing the speed with which the stomach empties, thus reducing the rate of absorption of carbohydrates.

In many ways, what we drink is more important than what we eat! The stomach empties liquids rapidly, rendering them suitable for quick absorption, and carbohydrate containing liquids have an extremely high glycemic index, producing rapid absorption and high blood glucose levels. As has been stated, a can of Coke contains nine to ten teaspoons of sugar. Conversely, if pure water, or a calorie-free drink, is taken, it has the effect of diluting the content of the stomach and slowing down the absorption of solid foods. Therefore, water, at least eight glasses a day, is recommended.

Beer has a high glycemic index as a result of its maltose content, which makes it even worse than table sugar. Wine and whiskey are safer bets because of the grains from which they are made, from different crops and vegetables. Red wine, in particular, has been shown to be healthy with its proven cardiac benefits. Coffee can be good; however, the caffeine content does stimulate the stomach to secrete acid and thereby increases the rate of digestion. This has the same effect on gastric emptying, and it may increase appetite. Tea also contains a considerable amount of caffeine and may be useful in the prevention of cardiac disease and even conditions such as prostate cancer. According to the protagonist of the South Beach diet, wine is less damaging than white bread, as its effect is less fattening. Barley, rye, and wheat, pure cereal grains, have glycemic indexes of 36%, 48%, and 59%, respectively. Most dairy foods have relatively low glycemic indexes, that for low-fat yogurt being only 20%, milk 39%, and fat-free milk 46%. Ice cream, perhaps unfortunately, has a glycemic index of 87%.

The glycemic index of fruits varies from 32% for cherries to 103% for watermelons. Grapefruit, peaches, oranges, and pears have a glycemic index of less than 50%; bananas and pineapples are much higher, being 89 and 94% respectively. The indexes of legumes vary, from 23% for soybeans to 70% for canned baked beans. Vegetables range from sweet potatoes at 63%, carrots at 70%, mashed potatoes at 100%, fries at 107%, to baked potatoes at 158%. With regard to simple sugars, the index for glucose is 137%; maltose, a major constituent of beer, 150%; lactose 92%; but fructose is only 32%. The following vegetables have a glycemic index of less than 20%: artichokes, asparagus, broccoli, Brussels sprouts, cabbage, cauliflower, celery, cucumbers, kale, mustard greens, spinach, peppers, and green beans; all of these vegetables are green in color. Turnips, mushrooms, and nuts also have a healthy, low glycemic index.

Vegetables are healthier than fruit, particularly green vegetables. Fruit juice could be even worse for your health than drinking cola and lemonade. A study of thirteen thousand adults published in the Journal of the American Medical Association in 2019 found that a 12-ounce glass of juice a day could increase early death by almost a quarter. Experts have said that the fructose content of such drinks could be driving up insulin resistance and stimulating hormones that promote fat deposition around the waist. Both can lead to a greater incidence of heart disease and diabetes. This study has shown, for the first time, that 100-percent fruit juices are very damaging to health. A daily glass of soda, such as cola, was linked to a 6% increased risk of early death over a sixyear period. In contrast, an extra fruit juice of the same volume was linked to a 24% rise in premature mortality in the same period of time. The reason is that the major sugar in fruit juice is fructose, which has a higher glycemic index than glucose, which is the major sugar in cola, so it is absorbed more rapidly, ultimately producing insulin resistance, which is extremely damaging to life.

Low glycemic index foods minimize food cravings. Alcoholic drinks with the best glycemic index are red wine and whiskey; beer has the worst because of its maltose content. The South Beach diet advocates the following vegetables, all of which have a low glycemic index: tomatoes, lettuce, onions, green peppers, garlic, shallots, mustard greens, olives, and broccoli, but it bans potatoes.

The initial stage of weight loss for people on the South Beach diet, quoted at eight to twelve pounds over the first two weeks, is due to reduced carbohydrate intake, which results in a loss of water storage, thereafter weight loss slows. Proponents of the South Beach diet strongly recommend an exercise program. Many people take a brisk twenty-minute walk daily, which is good but can only be expected to burn about a hundred calories. The majority of benefit gained from exercise occurs in the first twenty minutes, and following heavy exercise the increased burning of energy can occur for several hours. Weight training has many benefits; it improves muscle-to-fat ratio, increases metabolism, and promotes the body to burn fuel faster, even when sleeping. Increasing lean body mass—that is, body weight from muscle—is a positive benefit from weightlifting. Rapid, repeated weightlifting, even with light weights, as in body pump training, is a very useful form of exercise. Furthermore, exercise lowers blood pressure, increases good cholesterol, and other additions to a healthy diet, fish oil capsules and testosterone gel, have been recommended but without a lot of scientific proof of their efficacy.

The Ornish diet, which is high in fiber and low in fat, claims that heart disease can be reversed. The diet, like the preceding lowcarbohydrate diets, has been heavily promoted. Another lowcarbohydrate diet is the Protein Power Eades diet, which depends on the rationale that eating high protein and low fat adds to lean body mass and does not stimulate insulin; therefore, the overall effect is a slimmer and healthier body.

To increase longevity and long-term health, we are looking for a long-term, indeed lifelong, approach to diet. It has to be said that most diets ultimately fail. Even in the short term, most people tend to stray away from the specific diet and while being disillusioned return to their old bad eating habits. It has also been suggested that one reason why diets fail is that they create too much personal thought about food and what the subject is going to eat, and this tends to stimulate appetite. Another reason for failure is that people temporize on diets, thinking that a six-week crash diet will produce their desired effect, which, even if they managed to achieve it, is soon lost and reversed when the short period of dieting is over. It is safe to say that so much emphasis has been placed on diets and new diets through the media, television, and magazines that if any of these was highly successful in the long term, we would not now be facing such a massive increase in the number of obese people in the population.

All of the diets I have described places emphasis on drinking large amounts of water, at least eight glasses per day. That's a lot, but drink as much as you can!

There is a weight-loss program that is now thirty years old that depends upon what is described not so much as a diet as "natural hygiene." The basic concept and foundation of natural hygiene is that the body is always striving for health, which is achieved by continuously cleansing itself of deleterious waste material. It is not achieved by drinking water alone. According to the proponents of natural hygiene, high-water-content foods are the key. These are essentially vegetables, which not only contain large amounts of water, but all of the essential vitamins and minerals that have developed as a necessity for healthy life through the evolutionary process.

In those groups of people in the world already referred to who live extraordinarily long lives while maintaining good health, there is no obesity, and they live amazingly disease-free lives. It is claimed that they are free of heart disease and cancer. Their diet is essentially comprised of fruits and vegetables. The countries to which I am referring are the Abkhazians of Russia, the Vikabanbans of Ecuador, and the Hunzukuts of Pakistan.

Another important dietary factor is salt. Salt is added to most fast foods, bread, biscuits, and desserts. If taken in excess, it causes an increase in blood pressure. Therefore, my advice is not to add salt to your food.

I make no apology for placing such emphasis on diet. As stated, we are what we eat, and eating the right sort of diet is extremely important. Of the diets described, the South Beach probably offers the best chance of long-term adherence and longterm benefit. Simple reminders like eating green vegetables, white meat and fish, and drinking plenty of fluid cannot be overemphasized. This is the most important step that you can take to prolong your life, particularly if you combine it with regular exercise.

In summary, some calories are worth more than others. We are inducing our bodies to produce more insulin by present-day diets. One in seven deaths are now due to poor diet, and it is a worldwide problem. In the 1950s, looking at films and newsreels, everyone was slim. Then supermarkets sprung up, fast food and snacks were becoming popular, and so a new shape of man developed. A recent study showed that people who eat ultraprocessed food take in five hundred more calories per day than when they eat normally processed food. It is now realized that it is sugar, which is deadly. When fat was blamed, there was never any evidence for it, and it was not realized that sugar and insulin were responsible. If insulin levels are high, you are storing fat, and that is the problem underlying the current epidemic of obesity.

Chapter 17
Supermarkets: The Food We Buy

The increasing disparity in the range of incomes in the Western democracies has become a serious cause for concern, and there is evidence that those in higher income brackets live longer. This also appears to correlate with the level of education of the individual. All of us spend a significant part of our lives in the supermarket, and it is what we buy there, and how much we spend, that provides the basis for our diet and our health.

The last fifty years has brought about change, from shopping daily at the small, specialized corner shop, to buying groceries weekly from the supermarket. It is important to be careful about the consumption of foods bought from the supermarkets. For example, more fat is found in three slices of bread than in a calorierich Mars bar. Some breakfast cereals contain more than 15% fat, and some bestselling ready-made meals have more than triple the fat of other similar products. The amount of fat in pizzas can vary from 15 to 4%. Supermarkets provide often unchallenging comfort cuisine, rows and rows of ready-made foods from chicken potpies to sponge cakes that once would have been made at home. These products contain palm oil emulsifiers, hydrogenated vegetable oil, and a bewildering array of additives. These are used partly to ensure that foods last longer, taste better, and cost less. Fat is abundant, cheap, and can prolong the shelf life of products, adding an attractive texture. The result, over the past few decades, has been rising fat contents in many of the most popular foods.

Prolonged product longevity is an issue here. For example, a homemade lemon cake containing 10% fat would be stale and inedible after two or three days, while a supermarket cake with 20% fat tastes the same in three months as it does on the day you buy it. Fat emulsifiers are based on the chemistry that came out of the soap industry. They make fat more palatable. The result is that some breads contain 12% fat, whereas, in contrast, full-fat milk contains only 4%. According to the Atkins philosophy, this might not seem to be so important, but in all probability it is, and possibly extremely so. The reason being that trans fatty acids from hydrogenated vegetable fat used in cakes, cookies, and margarine are in themselves a health risk. Trans fatty acids cannot properly be digested, and the body simply stores them. There is evidence that trans fatty acids are involved in the formation of cholesterol deposits in the blood vessels in diabetes and obesity. On the other hand, monounsaturated fats, such as those found in avocados and nuts, are believed to be beneficial in moderation, possibly protecting against heart disease.

It may be, therefore, that the obesity revolution is not the responsibility of the consumer, but is contributed to, to some significant extent, by supermarkets, which control about 90% of food consumption. Supermarkets are presently going some way to provide healthy alternatives, and the labeling of energy content in food is increasingly being practiced. In the United Kingdom, the House of Commons select committee has recently criticized the food industry for not doing enough to promote healthy foods. They are introducing a traffic-light-system policy for labeling foods, those with increasing caloric intake being in the red zone.

A study reported in July 2004 involved 126 nutrition professionals with the American Dietetic Association, including sport nutritionists, cookbook and nutrition book authors, heads of hospital wellness programs, university weight loss researchers, and many dietitians in private practice. These national obesity researchers agreed that we cannot afford to allow the overweight population to increase over the next twenty years as it has over the last equivalent period. It has emphasized that a strategy must be formulated to prevent the one to two pounds that the average American gains each year. About 65% of adults in the US now weigh too much. This study determined the following major obstacles:

1. Most people do not have a realistic index of portion sizes. Restaurants contribute to the problem with portions that are at least twice the recommended serving size.
2. Children don't change bad eating habits for good; instead, they choose food they adhere to in the short term only and then revert to their previous eating habits.
3. Most people consider exercise a drudgery and rarely stay with exercise program.
4. There is a large reluctance to change eating habits as people become addicted to their favorite foods.
5. People fail to realize that there is no such thing as a miracle diet. What the overweight want to hear is that losing weight is quick, easy, miraculous and involves little effort. No such system exists.

The nutritionists in this study felt that a big problem was that activity had been squeezed out of people's lives by modern technology. Moving from cars, to desks, to television screens and computers has ruled exercise out of most people's way of existence.

Chapter 18
Dementia

A major cause of death that is rapidly increasing in its prevalence is dementia, and dietary factors are major contributory factors hereto. Dementia describes symptoms of memory loss, particularly short-term memory difficulties with thinking, problem solving, and carrying out day-to-day activities. These symptoms are associated with depressed mood, reduced activity, and withdrawal from work and social activities.

Alzheimer's disease is the major cause of dementia, which may also be due to cardiovascular disease that is associated with heart disease and arteriosclerosis, and there are other causes. Worldwide, about forty-seven million people suffer from dementia. The estimated proportion of the general population aged sixty and over with dementia is about 7%, a figure which increases with increasing age. These numbers have been assessed to almost double in the next twenty years. It is not an inevitable consequence of aging. Many people over the age of one hundred are alert, clear thinking, and have excellent recall.

The risk factors for dementia are those common to other major killers like heart disease, stroke, and some cancers, all of which relate to a major extent to diet. Seven lifestyle factors throughout middle age have a significant influence on the risk of developing dementia later in life. These are: weight, diet, exercise, cholesterol levels, blood sugar and diabetes, hypertension, and smoking. In a large study in France, people over the age of sixty-five were tested for these seven parameters and then monitored for an average of eight and a half years. For every single item of the seven factors, for those who passed as healthy, the risk of developing dementia went down by 10% each. The study clearly demonstrates the link between cardiovascular health and the resilience of the brain with exactly the same key triggering factors as those that occur with the other major killers. Thus, the risk of dementia can be reduced by living a healthy lifestyle and eating the right items of food. Age remains a factor in the equation, but the risk can be reduced, and age, per se, is not the major or even an essential factor in developing dementia. What is good for the heart, therefore, is good for the brain. The risk factors are present for many years and begin in early life, so it is never too early to modify lifestyle accordingly and take the right steps to reduce the risk. This includes taking steady exercise, staying mentally active, and being socially engaged.

Eating an appropriate diet is therefore an essential and major factor in maintaining brain function. This is a more significant factor than genetics, which contributes 10%. Therefore, 90% is down to lifestyle, and in this situation lifestyle is down to diet, and diet is essential for adequate genetic function. Interestingly, the dietary factors that contribute to the maintenance of brain function are essentially those that have been discussed in terms of cardiovascular disease and diabetes. There are additional essential requirements for the more complex brain. It is vulnerable to a poor diet, brain cells continuously turn over, and the breakdown of proteins and amino acids help to form new brain cells. In addition to protein, vegetables, fruit, and whole grains supply energy to the cells. Omega-3 and, to a lesser extent, omega-6 fatty acids contribute to the structure of cellular linings. Trans fats found in large amounts in fast foods again are bad news here, as are refined sugars. We are eating more fast foods rich in the latter, and these are contributing to the rapid increase in cognitive disorders and Alzheimer's disease.

The brain-healthy diet should contain white meat, fish, vegetables and a good fluid intake, but not high-calorie sugary drinks. Some vitamins are essential for the brain, particularly the antioxidants vitamins A, C, and E. Vitamin A is wholesome in carrots, vitamin E, which increases the delivery of oxygen to brain cells, is present in peppers and broccoli, and vitamin C can be found in berries and citrus fruit. The water-soluble B vitamins, vitamin B12, folate, and vitamin B6, are also essential stimulants of brain cellular function.

Plants contain a lot of antioxidants that prevent inflammation. Onions, garlic, and fresh herbs are a great source, just as they are in preventing cardiovascular disease.

People asked me, "What about coffee?" That has been controversial, some suggesting an increased incidence of pancreatic cancer, though hard evidence for this is lacking. Coffee is, however, rich in antioxidants, and the caffeine is a stimulant to the brain. The choice of protein is important and directly corresponds to that recommended for vascular disease. Red meat and rich dairy products such as high-cream milk and cheese contain saturated fats and should be avoided; skimmed milk is better, and you will easily get used to it as a replacement for whole milk. I have avoided mentioning butter, because a source of some fat is essential. The argument between butter and margarine continues essentially unresolved. Replace red meat with chicken, turkey, lean pork, and fish. Salmon is an excellent source of protein and is very rich in omega-3.

Forbidden in the 1950s to the 1970s, eggs with high cholesterol content in the yolks have over the years been favorably reappraised. They are rich in protein and omega-3 fatty acids and other antioxidants. Two to three eggs per week are probably quite beneficial, but the question remains controversial. The role of fat also remains controversial. Too much saturated fat undoubtedly increases the risk of heart disease, type 2 diabetes, and dementia. A large study has shown that those eating the most saturated fat have four times the risk of cognitive deterioration compared to those on the lowest amount. Cheese may be eaten sparingly.

Today, well over 50% of new cases of dementia either have a vascular or a mixed vascular/Alzheimer's cause. Structured lifestyle interventions over time can dramatically diminish cognitive decline. At least 40% of dementia is preventable. Practical changes to diet, stress levels, sleep routine, and activity with social interaction can slow down its progress. Just twenty minutes of brisk walking per day can facilitate information processing and memory function.

Looking to the future, because vascular disease can play such a major role in cognitive decline, it has recently been suggested that an ultrasound scan of the blood vessels in the neck can predict dementia ten years before the symptoms appear. Measuring the degree of arterial impairment through the carotid arteries in the neck can predict vascular damage to the brain, which impairs memory and thinking skills. Vascular disease in the neck due to hypertension can produce damage to very small, fragile vessels that supply the brain, often causing small bleeds, which can destroy brain cells, causing memory and thinking problems and even minor strokes. Three thousand people were studied over a fifteen-year period, with a measurement of their high-intensity carotid pulse at the beginning of the study and an assessment of their cognitive capacities at the end. Those with carotid artery disease and a high-intensity pulse were 50% more likely to have accelerated cognitive decline. This is an easily measurable and potentially treatable cause of cognitive decline in middle-aged individuals that can be spotted in advance and corrected. No major breakthroughs have been made in the treatment of established dementia.

In Alzheimer's disease there is a build up of sticky amyloid plaques in the brain, which prevent neurons from communicating. This can occur for up to twenty years before any symptoms show. Researchers from Washington University Medical School have in August 2019, described a blood test which is 94% accurate in detecting Alzheimer's disease many years before people develop memory loss and confusion. This could prove to be fundamentally important, not only in the detection, but ultimately in the treatment of this the major killing disease of the elderly.

Chapter 19
Sleep

We spend one-third of our lives sleeping, but is it important to health? Sleep matters for maintaining good health. There is little firm and irrevocable evidence on how long we should sleep, but information is being gathered to show that sleep influences the risk of dementia.

As we age, our circadian sleep cycles shorten, and many become sleepless in old age, but super-agers sleep for at least eight hours at night, and a nap in the daytime helps relieve stress. During sleep, toxins are cleared from the brain and cells repair and grow. A buildup of toxins in the brain leads to inflammation, which can destroy blood vessels and interfere with cellular function. Sleep improves cellular mechanisms and can improve memory, short-term memory, which tends to be compromised by aging. Impaired sleep patterns occur with the early symptoms of dementia and increase as the disease progresses. Removal of toxins from the brain during sleep may prevent the buildup of amyloid plaques that destroy brain cells in Alzheimer's disease. Interrupted sleep patterns that occur with sleep apnea, anxiety, and depression are associated with a higher risk of dementia. Sleeping less at night seems to affect the hormonal patterns that regulate hunger and satiety, leading to obesity, further sleep apnea, and a higher incidence of dementia.

Throughout life, seven to nine hours of sleep at night seems optimal. Deep-sleep and restorative slow-wave sleep patterns tend to reduce with age. Sleep can also be interrupted by painful conditions such as joint and back disease, and there is a high incidence of gastroesophageal reflux disease, which is exacerbated by eating shortly before retiring.

A regular sleep rhythm is good. Heavy eating or intense exercise should be avoided late at night, as these stimulate metabolism. The bedroom should be dark and silent. Today, so many are using social media, reading emails, and looking at phones throughout the night, which are clearly obstructive to normal sleep. Caffeine in coffee and tea should be avoided close to sleeping. Alcohol may induce sleep, but ultimately acts as a stimulus, causing frequent awakening.

Sleeping pills can certainly work but should be avoided if possible. They tend not to work in the long term and can be addictive. Melatonin, the sleep hormone, taken in tablet form is widely used, and natural levels become depleted with age. It can be helpful particularly to the elderly. There are many over-the-counter herbal remedies such as Valerian and passion flower but, on the whole, these are of little value.

Sleep, therefore, is part of the equation in maintaining a long and healthy life. It isn't just important for replenishing energy levels. Scientists increasingly believe it affects brain function in the long term and influences the risk of dementia and Parkinson's disease.

Chapter 20
What to do in Retirement?

Super-agers tend to have a unique personality profile, highlighting optimism, resilience, and perseverance, some of which can be developed.

Put the stress of your job behind you. The workplace in general has become more bureaucratic, demanding, threatening, and is riddled with professional jealousy. Put your work behind you and do something new that you enjoy and that is not stressful or competitive. Enthuse in the hobbies that you can become passionate about. Do some work, if this interests you, does not stress you, and is not competitive. Choose a form of exercise that you like, from walking the dog to swimming, running, or playing golf, tennis, or another sport. Do something that you enjoy, and do not regard it as a chore or an irreversible commitment.

Don't look back on your earlier life; look forward. Retrospection creates resentfulness, unhappiness, and depression. These latter feelings create stress and can lead to heart attack and stroke. Take the opportunity to learn new things or go to classes and mix with others through societies that are of interest to you. Getting out of the house is important, even going to the coffee bar or library. Learning a new language or discipline will become a very positive factor in your life. It is good to be friends with people of all ages and all walks of life. Exchanging common interests with people of variable age is good, if it is on an equal exchange of information basis. Make an impression by dressing smartly, looking presentable, and not letting standards slip. This will create a more positive response to you from others. When communicating with others, pay attention all the time; it will create mutual respect. Volunteer for activities, provided you enjoy it, it is not stressful, and people don't abuse your goodwill. Spending most of the day sitting in front of the television is bad and will damage your overall attitude to life and your positivity.

Chapter 21
Drugs and Longevity

It has been demonstrated in recent years that several medications can prolong life. Anti-hypertensive drugs are plentiful and effective in reducing the risk of death from heart attacks and strokes. Chemotherapy drugs, though extremely toxic, can prolong life and even cure some forms of cancer. The statins are a widely used group of drugs that effectively reduce cholesterol and reduce deaths from heart attacks and strokes.

New drugs are also being developed; importantly, the lipoprotein lipase enhancers, which could further substantially cut the risk of disease in those taking statins. These drugs effectively reduce triglyceride fats in the blood. They are thought to have the potential for cutting the risk of heart attacks and angina by 40% and type 2 diabetes by 30%. In Great Britain, statins are taken by six million people and are thought to save about eight thousand lives per year. The new drugs, the lipoprotein lipase enhancers, are thought to improve blood glucose control in diabetics.

Another new drug, leucoserin, stimulates some brain cells called PDMC, neurons that control appetite. These cells become less efficient with increasing age, and this may contribute to the "middle-age spread." It has been shown in a large clinical trial in the United States that those taking the drug lost an average of 9 lbs. 3 oz. in one year, compared with three pounds in those on diet alone. Those treated by the drug kept their weight off for at least three years. Community weight-loss groups do claim that they can achieve similar weight loss, and the above drug is expensive. There were no adverse cardiological or other side effects from it compared with alternative existing drug therapy for obesity.

It has been shown that the accumulation of senescent cells in the body and brain is linked to aging, frailty, joint problems, arthritis, Alzheimer's, and Parkinson's disease. These senescent cells, also called zombie cells, are not completely dead and so are not cleared from the body, but they are incapable of repair and waste clearance, so the body deteriorates in their presence. Animal studies have shown that removing these cells reverses the aging process, extends life expectancy, and restores youthfulness. Recently, scientists in the United States have developed a drug that can sweep away these deficient cells. A small three-week trial on fourteen patients showed that the drug appeared safe. The participants were able to walk faster, get up from the chair better, and had improved cognition. The senior author on this study, James Kirkland of the Mayo Clinic, published this data in the Lancet, stating, "This is a glimmer of light that might actually work. The results are impressive, and all fourteen patients got improved functional ability."

There are at least twenty conditions in which senescent cells are implicated. The above was an initial study, and other human studies are moving fast. This study showed that the drug began clearing out senescent cells within just thirty minutes, and then, within twenty-four hours, all of the dying cells were gone. An improvement in breathing has also been shown with this drug in patients suffering from pulmonary fibrosis.

It is now suspected that many of the killing diseases associated with aging share common mechanisms, so that drugs that target senescent cells or modify the characteristics may represent a new avenue of treatment for other diseases of aging in the future. The scientists from the Mayo Clinic now believe that the aging process itself is associated with the buildup of senescent cells and is responsible for major conditions such as Alzheimer's disease, Parkinson's disease, arthritis, cancer, heart disease, and diabetes, and they now have potentially found a way to turn them off.

These and other new antiaging drugs, called serolytics, are being investigated, unlike previous drug studies, collectively on multiple diseases and are assessed on their ability to prevent or alleviate most age-related illnesses and frailty. Six trials are currently underway, and more are being set up. If successful, they estimate that drugs that slow down the aging process could be ready for general usage by 2022. In mice, the drugs extend lifespan by 36%, the equivalent of adding about thirty years to the life of the human, and, crucially, the animals remained in good health. Aging itself is currently the highest identifiable risk factor for most of the chronic killing diseases, and if you get one of these, you're likely to get others.

It is very likely that the semaglutides, the weight reducing drugs like Wegovy and Ozempic will in the long term be shown to increase life expectancy. Thus, there are great possibilities, in the near future, for an increase in longevity, but along with the marathon of life, the factors outlined herein should be adhered to as closely as possible.

Chapter 22
Deaths from Trauma

A major, and often unavoidable, cause of death, particularly in the young, is trauma. There are many causes of major trauma, blunt and penetrating, including falls, motor vehicle accidents, stabbings, and gunshot wounds. In the United States, most deaths caused by penetrating trauma occur in urban areas, and 82% of these deaths are caused by firearms. In the UK, where there are strong restrictive laws on the possession of firearms, there has been a disturbingly huge increase in deaths from stabbing. It has been estimated that unintentional and intentional injuries accounted for 6% and 3%, respectively, of all deaths.

The leading causes of posttraumatic death are blunt trauma, motor vehicle accidents, and falls, followed by penetrating trauma such as stabbings and gunshot wounds. Many injuries are due to suicide. Occupational and sports injuries contribute to these numbers.

By identifying risk factors present within the community and creating solutions to decrease the incidence of injury, trauma referral systems and major trauma centers may help to improve the overall health of the population. Injury prevention strategies are commonly used to prevent injuries to children. These generally involve educating the general public about specific risk factors and developing strategies to avoid and reduce injuries. Government strategies, such as compulsory use of seatbelts, child car seats, motorcycle helmets, and alcohol restriction, contribute to a reduction in injuries. A factor of concern is drugs, which contribute substantially to motor vehicle accidents. Prescription drugs such as hydrocodone derivatives and benzodiazepines are at the risk of increasing motor vehicle accidents, particularly in the elderly. Throughout the world, deaths from injuries are most common in Russia, central Africa, and Indonesia.

These factors result in trauma being the sixth leading cause of death and the fifth leading cause of disability worldwide. Sixty-eight percent of traumatic injuries occur in males. Younger people, being more active, are prone to acute traumatic injuries, while elderly persons are more likely to die from the injuries they sustain. Children are much more prone to road traffic accidents and drowning. Thus, accidents are the leading cause of death in children between the ages of one and fourteen. In the United States, about sixteen million children go to emergency departments due to some form of injury every year.

CHAPTER 23
SUICIDE

Risk factors for suicide are mental disorders that include depression, bipolar disorder, schizophrenia, personality disorders, and substance abuse, including alcoholism. Predisposing factors are stressful situations such as financial difficulties, divorce, and problems in the workplace. Easy access to firearms, drugs, and poisons enable easy suicide. Methods of suicide vary according to the access to the above.

Suicides resulted in 828,000 global deaths in 2015, and the numbers are increasing annually, making suicide the tenth leading cause of death worldwide; that is half a percent of the world population. Suicides are more likely to occur in third-world countries, and rates are globally higher in males than females. The highest incidence is in those over the age of seventy, but there is a smaller peak between fifteen and thirty years of age. Suicide is encouraged as a form of terrorism, which results in mass murder in some communities. Euthanasia is related to suicide but is less common and is illegal in most countries. Many attempted suicides are incomplete. Veterans who frequently suffer from posttraumatic stress disorder are at higher risk, and genetics play a role in suicidal behavior.

There is no known unifying, underlying cause for either suicide or depression. It is, however, believed to result from an interplay of behavioral, socio-environmental, and psychiatric factors. Low levels of a biochemical compound, designated BDNF, are both directly associated with suicide and indirectly connected through its role in major depression, posttraumatic stress disorder, schizophrenia, and obsessive-compulsive disorder. Changes in the brain are detectable in those dying from suicide. The chemical serotonin is low in many who died as a result of suicide. There are also genetic factors involved.

Suicide rates vary widely between different countries, being highest in Russia, China, India, and Pakistan. Rates of deaths per hundred thousand are: Australia (8.6), Canada (11.1), China (12.7), India (23.2), United Kingdom (7.6), United States (11.4), and South Korea (28.9). There are about 45,000 deaths per year from suicide in the United States, and about 650,000 are seen in emergency rooms yearly due to attempted suicide. In Western countries, males exceed females by about 1.8 to 1, though in China it is more common in females. There is a marked increase in the incidence of suicide among transgender, lesbian, gay, and bisexual people. Transgender individuals are reported to have a 40% incidence of attempted suicide. Physician-assisted suicide is a highly controversial issue, being illegal in most Western countries.

CHAPTER 24
THE UNPREDICTABLE

Unpredictable factors that can have an influence on longevity are:

WRECKS
- Wars
- Refugees
- Economics
- Climate
- Kings and dictators
- Suicide

There are many factors that are unpredictable in their effect on longevity but have in the past had a major impact and may do so in the future. By far the most costly war in terms of human life was World War II, in which the total number of fatalities, including battle deaths and civilians of all countries, has been estimated at seventy million. Adult males have always tended to be those subject to the greatest mortality. In the Paraguayan War of 1864 to 1870 against Brazil, Argentina, and Uruguay, Paraguay's population was reduced from 407,000 to 221,000 survivors, of whom fewer than 30,000 were adult males. It goes without saying that war has been a major killer since the beginning of recorded history. It is stated in the Bible that there will always be wars and rumors of wars, and this so far has proved to be true. It has been estimated that between 350 million and more than 750 million people have died in wars. Historically, the Qing conquest of the Ming Empire thousands of years ago caused in excess of 25 million deaths; the Mongol conquests led to 35 million deaths in total. John F. Kennedy famously stated, "Mankind must put an end to war before war puts an end to mankind."

In the modern era, ever increasingly deadly technology and a booming world population, amounting to overpopulation, could bring about a nuclear war and an unprecedented number of deaths.

During their lives, many people have been displaced and forced to cross national boundaries; sometimes, large-scale migration occurs as a result of wars or economic deprivation. In 1917, one and a half million people fled the Russian Revolution, which brought in communism. Recently in the Middle East, millions have fled Syria, and the communist regime in Venezuela completely destroyed what was a vibrant economy and has led to millions fleeing that country. The first half of the twentieth century brought about the migration across national boundaries in Europe of millions of refugees during and after two world wars. During 2017, it has been estimated that 25.4 million people were forcibly displaced from their countries of origin. Displacement tends to be a long-lasting situation for most, which totally changed their lifestyle, their economic situation, their diet, their health, and, along with severe stress imposed upon them, resulted in a reduction in life expectancy.

Refugees typically report poorer health than the nonimmigrant population. Posttraumatic stress disorder and depression are very common and severely impede the functionality of these people. Suicide rates are also high in refugees.

Kings and dictators have executed millions throughout history. Most recently, Stalin killed twenty-one million of his own people, Hitler killed millions, and now Assad has exterminated millions of Syrians.

Major economic decline can produce humanitarian crises and deaths on the large scale. As a result of the political crisis in Venezuela, more than three million have fled their country. Foreign aid is blocked at the borders, and starvation is prevalent in the remaining population. More than a thousand Caritas neighborhood kitchens are currently operating at full capacity. Food aid and nutritional support for malnourished children is badly needed. The richer middle class has long left the country. Few people have money, as the inflation rate increases exponentially. Few medicines are available to the population. More than one and a half million Venezuelans have entered Columbia. Thousands continue to cross the border every day, and reception capacities are greatly overstretched. Clearly, there are many unforeseen factors that can greatly affect lifestyle and longevity.

In the near future, we may be facing a major threat from climate change. Climate change occurs when changes in the Earth's climate system result in different weather patterns. Cyclical ocean patterns change, such as the El Nino southern oscillation, which can produce short-term climate changes. Catastrophic events like the collision of a large meteorite into the Gulf of Mexico led to the extermination of the dinosaurs. Human activities are currently being blamed for the present-day global warming. The increased use of fossil fuels is thought to be the major factor, and this produces at least, on a theoretical basis, major threats to lifestyle and longevity.

CHAPTER 25
CONCLUSIONS—THE BOTTOM LINE

A recent study published in the Lancet has stated that poor diet is now a bigger risk to life than smoking. With the reduced number of smokers and the fast escalation of fast food and sugary drinks consumption, diet is now to blame for most early deaths. Approximately one in six deaths is now linked to unhealthy eating. Low intake of vegetables, whole grains, fiber, and fruit are the biggest problems. Excess consumption of processed meat, salt, and sugary drinks is the main problem. Education is required to guide families towards healthy eating.

Researchers from the University of Washington have stated that the vast majority of diet-related deaths are due to heart disease, followed by cancer and type 2 diabetes. Campaigns on the reduction of salt consumption have lost momentum. Ninety percent of adults fail to eat the recommended amount of fiber. Meanwhile, junk food is booming, with more and more takeouts opening, and about 50% of children are now overweight. The emphasis should be positive, stressing the importance of healthy foods rather than directly condemning fast foods.

In the US, it has been estimated that 171 deaths per hundred thousand people per year are linked to diets, and 127 per hundred thousand in the UK. This is in marked contrast to 900 per hundred thousand in Afghanistan. Israel, France, and Spain had the lowest diet-related death rates in the world, with 89 per hundred thousand. Most of these are avoidable deaths. The initial, most clear, step is to reduce sugar intake. The advice to be given about alcohol consumption is difficult, as it remains controversial. The results of a ten-year study from Oxford and a Chinese university on 160,000 patients reported a 15% increase in stroke in people who drank alcohol.

Over recent years, food has gone from being a limited and often scarce source to a flavorsome and often exotic experience. Restaurants have greatly increased in their numbers and variety; takeouts and even home deliveries have also ballooned. Half the money spent on food in the US is spent in restaurants. Relatively speaking, food has become much less expensive. Lower socioeconomic groups used to have to spend more than half of their income on food, whereas now, about 10% of the family income goes in that direction. Malnutrition, which affected about half the world's population, is now fortunately much rarer, affecting about 10%. Farming efficiency has greatly improved, along with refrigeration and globalization of virtually all foods.

Despite these improvements, the fast-food revolution has greatly undermined public health, and poor diets now kill one in six people. This is the new form of malnutrition, piling in the calories while reducing the essential nutrients. We are eating many more calories than our predecessors, in front of our computers and social media devices. It has been estimated that the average person in the US and UK eats five hundred calories per day more than they did in the 1960s, and these are the wrong sort of calories, which is heavily loaded with simple carbohydrates and low on protein.

The average adult today eats 120 grams of vegetables per day, compared with 450 grams fifty years ago. It is amazing to consider that McDonald's is now a worldwide company, and a new branch of Domino's Pizza opens somewhere in the world every seven hours. Double burgers contain bacon and cheese, as well as extra carbohydrates being inserted into the bread, and a milkshake can contain a thousand calories. Bread is now saturated in sugar, salt, and preservatives to improve its taste and prolong its life. The processed foods yield much greater profits than whole foods, and there is less waste. Consequently, much more is spent on advertising them. Our overall food culture needs to change, with better education and governmental intervention to promote healthier eating.

Although it passes by unperceptively, with apparently everincreasing speed, life is a marathon, not a hundred-yard dash. Many will die in childhood or their twenties and thirties from malignancies, trauma, and suicide, but overall, statistically, there are things that can be done to increase your longevity, and most of these relate to diet and, of course, not smoking.

The disease that is increasing most in prevalence is Type-2 diabetes, which leads to heart disease, blindness, kidney failure, nerve damage, and amputation of the lower limbs. There has been up to a tenfold increase in the incidence of diabetes in Western countries in the last thirty or forty years, and it is all related to diet, and sugar is the major enemy.

You should start by cutting out potatoes, pasta, bread, cakes, and drinks containing sugar. A general practitioner, David Unwin, in Southport, England, has had remarkable success with the program that he set up in his practice. In 1986, he had fifty-seven patients in his practice with type 2 diabetes. Thirty years on, he had 470, and it was developing at a much younger age. Following his advice, 40% of these patients have reversed their diabetes completely, and the blood pressure, cholesterol, and liver function of all improved. Coincidently, they have lost an average of twenty pounds in weight in twenty months.

Unwin's strategy follows the principles outlined in this book. There are seven rules to his successful plan:

1. Reduce or eliminate sugar and starch in carbohydrate foods. These include breakfast cereals, bread, pasta, white potatoes, rice, couscous, crackers, oats, cakes, sweets, milk chocolate, fruit juice, fizzy drinks, and cordials, which carbohydrates.
2. Eat plenty of vegetables at each meal, using nonstarchy and salad vegetable such as broccoli, courgettes, green beans, aubergines (eggplant), and reduce your consumption of root vegetables.
3. Eat good fats. Include oily fish, olive oil, coconut oil, avocado, and a minimal amount of animal fats. You can eat nuts and some cheeses, but they are calories.
4. Don't eat too much fruit, and avoid bananas, mango, pineapples, and fruits which are high in sugar and have a high glycemic index.

5. Eat a lot of protein, the best forms of which are white meat, chicken, turkey fowl, fish, and lean pork. Steak and red meats should be restricted to once a week.
6. Stop snacking. Fasting between meals and overnight helps to improve resistance; you can eat three meals a day.
7. Drink two liters of water each day, Zero-calorie drinks are also acceptable.

These are the principles that have now been shown to be sound and scientifically credible, though it may seem like an extreme example of eating to live rather than living to eat. Quality of life is important. The above parameters could be used as useful guidelines, but use some flexibility and it will give more enjoyment to eating. Simply put, I would advise eating green vegetables and white meat and fish as much as possible, while observing the dangers of eating too much of those items listed above that are prohibited. Also, exercise, try to walk ten thousand steps per day when you can. A useful little guide is the Fitbit, a small pen-sized electronic device attached to your clothes that quite accurately records steps climbed, miles walked, and calories burned.

Good luck in achieving a happy, healthy, and active long life.

SUGGESTED FURTHER READING

Agatston, A. *The South Beach Diet.* Rodale, 2003.

Andrews, S., et al. *Sugar Busters.* Vermillion, 2005.

Atkins, R.C. *Age-Defying Diet Revolution.* St. Martin's Press, 2000.

Atkins, R.C. *Atkins for Life.* St. Martin's Press, 2003.

Barnard, N. *Foods that Cause You to Lose Weight.* Avon, 2002.

Bailey, C. *The Eight-Week Blood Sugar Diet.* Short Books, 2019.

Christou, N.V. et al. "Surgery Decreases Long-term Mortality, Morbidity and Health Care Use in Morbidly Obese Patients." *Annual of Surgery,* 2004: 240, 416.

Estruch, R. et al. "Primary Prevention of Cardiovascular Disease with a Mediterranean Diet." *New England Journal of Medicine,* 2013: 368, 1279.

Fontana, L. et al. "Extending Healthy Lifespan." *Science,* 2010: 328, 321.

Gebel, K. et al. "Effect of Moderate to Vigorous Physical Activity on Mortality." *JAMA,* 2015: 175, 6.

Gillespie, S. *Britain's Diabetes Explosion.* British Heart Foundation, 2019.

Longo, V. *The Longevity Diet.* Penguin, 2016.

Martin, L.F. Obesity Surgery. McGraw Hill, 2004.

Olshansky, S.J. et al. "Decline in Life Expectancy in the United States in the 21st Century." *New England Journal of Medicine,* 2015: 352, 1138.

Ornish, D.M. et al. "Can Lifestyle Changes Reverse Coronary Atherosclerosis?" *Lancet,* 1990: 336, 129.

Samieri, C., "Lifestyle Factors Behind Dementia." *JAMA,* 2019.

Taylor, T.V. *Overcoming Obesity.* Vantage, New York. 2007.

Taylor, T.V. et al. *Upper Digestive Surgery,* Saunders, 2007.

Wilson, B. *The Way We Eat,* Basic Books, 2019.

www.ingramcontent.com/pod-product-compliance
Lightning Source LLC
Chambersburg PA
CBHW052033030426
42337CB00027B/4983